HEINERMAN'S

ENCYCLOPEDIA *of* HEALING JUICES

JOHN HEINERMAN

REWARD BOOKS
a member of
Penguin Group (USA)
New York

This book is a reference work based on research by the author. The opinions expressed herein are not necessarily those of or endorsed by the publisher. The directions stated in this book are in no way to be considered as a substitute for consultation with a duly licensed doctor.

The recipes contained in this book are to be followed exactly as written. The publisher is not responsible for your specific health or allergy needs that may require medical supervision. The publisher is not responsible for any adverse reactions to the recipes contained in this book.

✦ Reward Books
a member of
Penguin Group (USA) Inc.
375 Hudson Street
New York, NY 10014
www.penguin.com

Library of Congress Cataloging-in-Publication Data

Heinerman, John.
    Heinerman's encyclopedia of juice cures / John Heinerman.
       p.   cm.
    Includes index.
    ISBN 0-13-057571-2 (case)—ISBN 0-13-057548-8 (pbk.)
     1. Fruit juices.   2. Vegetable juices.   I. Title.
  RM255.H45   1994   94-2753
  613.2'6—dc20   CIP

Printed in the United States of America

20   19   18   17   16   15

XX   (paper)

Most Reward Books are available at special quantity discounts for bulk purchases for sales promotions, premiums, fund-raising, or educational use. Special books, or book excerpts, can also be created to fit specific needs.

For details, write: Special Markets, Penguin Group (USA) Inc., 375 Hudson Street, New York, New York 10014.

*Dedicated To
Joseph Smith, Jr., an American Prophet*

FOREWORD

I am impressed with this book. I read almost every word.

I have known and worked with John Heinerman for some years. He writes almost as fast as he talks. He is full of anecdotes about his subject and the people from whom he has learned so many things. He has been privileged to have been able to travel around the world. He does not seem to be afraid to talk to people about their habits and their methods of seeking health. He knows why plants, fruits, vegetables work, and the reader of this book will be surprised and impressed by how so many lowly fruits and vegetables can be so helpful to the ailing.

Most doctors are locked into the concept that only one, specific, unique drug should be used to treat one specific malady. One drug fits one disease. But Mother Nature does not work that way. Most herbs, vegetables, and fruits have a bi-directional ability. Some natural remedies will lower blood pressure if it is high, and the same substance will raise it if it is low. John Heinerman points out that cabbage, celery, and lettuce contain the ingredients that will stabilize the blood sugar levels, increasing it if it is down and lowering it if it is up. Sulfur seems to be the key element, but it must be combined with other vitamins. minerals, and alkaloids in order to do this for us. Combinations, not single entities, give the therapeutic benefits. The ancients, and now John Heinerman (not an ancient), knew this. We are privileged to have it laid out and organized so well in this book. It is full of Nature's truths and replete with John's famous stories of the benefits of juices. How come the Hunzas look so good? The answer is in these pages. I thought they were lying about their ages. No, they just look good at age 90 years or so. It is no secret and you can do the same for yourself if you follow John's juicing suggestions.

Most of us have forgotten how to chew (or cannot) well enough to break down the cell walls. If you have lost many teeth because of the impoverished American diet you have been eating all these years, your gums and false teeth may not be adequate to act as your own personal inexpensive juicer. Those lost teeth are a clue that you need fruits and vegetables for their hidden nutrients. You may have to buy a juicer. Juicing opens up the indigestible cellulose walls of plants so our bodies can reap those intracellular bounties. Some of the fiber that may be lost in the juicing process should be consumed for its benefits. John points this fact out by his suggestion as to which type of juicer to use.

This book tells you what to take for what conditions, and John gives you encouraging stories about people all over the world who have benefited from their use. He gives the amounts of the nutrients in each of the foods he has selected.

One way to find out if you are getting the proper amounts of minerals, especially the ones that are used by the body as electrolytes (sodium, potassium, chloride) is to take your own blood pressure every few days, and to evaluate your circulation by the temperature of your feet and hands. You should be able to notice that the veins on the backs of your hands have some blue blood flowing through them. The veins should continue to have some blood flowing through them as you elevate your hand up to your eye level. If you are drinking juices and your blood pressure is low (below 115/75), your hands and feet are cool, and the veins are flat at your nipple level, you should add more water to your juices.

If you get one of those standard 24 chemical analyses of your blood, you will be able to determine if your electrolytes are above or below the mean (the halfway point of the range). Most all fruits and vegetables have 20 to 100 times as much potassium as sodium. This is why vegetarians almost never have to worry about high blood pressure, as the sodium is more likely to be responsible for the elevation of the systolic pressure. Potassium will almost always lower the diastolic figure. If you take your blood pressure and it is low (below 115/60) you might want to add some table salt to your juice to bring up the systolic pressure. (Of course, talk to your doctor.)

John Heinerman is giving the public the opportunity to get healthy in a cheap, safe way. After all most of us are scared about the toxic drugs that medical doctors are taught to prescribe. They almost always have side-effects. The reader of this volume who is already on some medication might try these time-honored remedies while still taking the prescribed drugs, and then after a few weeks check with the doctor to see if a reduction in the dose might be appropriate.

John's description of his lusting after parsley struck a responsive chord with me. He tells about a hay fever attack that just would not go away. He spied some parsley in a cafeteria where he was staying, and had a sudden urge to eat a whole plate-full. His brain said "Go for it!" In a few minutes when it was digested his sneezing and rhinorrhea had completely stopped. I am involved with a program that encourages people to eat food that they like—exclusive of alcohol and sugar, of course. The body seems to know what is good for it at any certain time and sends a message to the brain to forage for that item. I need vitamin A, and will lust after carrots, squash, sweet potato, and steal parsley off other diner's plates. I assume it is because my skin is not perfect and my body knows I must get extra beta-carotene and vitamin A. John notes that parsley has a whopping 850 I.U. of vitamin A in ten sprigs of parsley. Everyday foods do possess wonderful healing properties to fight off illnesses and prolong our lives.

This book is full of cheerful information. It is hard to not get excited about the multiple uses of Mother Nature's bounty.

Sincerely,

Lendon H. Smith, MD

PREFACE

The idea or rather the *need* for writing a juice book came to me quite by accident. As much as I'd love to call it a stroke of inspiration, I honestly can't. Because, you see, it was more like a moment of complaint that began this whole arduous and challenging process.

I was speaking at one of numerous alternative health conventions that I'm invited to every year. The exhibit I was sitting at autographing books and answering people's questions happened to be right next to the booth of the most expensive juice machine on the market (not mentioned in this book, however).

A certain lady in her fifties had been patiently watching the carrot juice demonstration and inquired if the exhibitors had a juice book to sell. She was informed in rather abrupt terms that they didn't and that a book wasn't necessary to operate their machine.

She came over to where I was, visibly annoyed by the response she had just received. Seeing me free, she started off our conversation by asking rather loudly, "Why can't someone write a book about juicing that people like me can understand? Why can't I get the information I want when I need it the most?"

Then trailing off in her thoughts momentarily, she looked down on the table and saw my best-selling book, *Heinerman's Encyclopedia of Fruits, Vegetables and Herbs*. Recognizing me from my lectures she had attended earlier that day, she asked in an off-handed manner: "Why don't *you* write a book on juicing? At least it would tell me what I want to know!" Our conversation after that was confined to her own personal health problems. Her complaint stuck in my mind for some reason. It just wouldn't let go. Not that I was terribly anxious to write another health book mind you, but the challenge just seemed to sit there all alone, somehow waiting to be accepted by me.

Not too long after this, in a phone conversation with my good friend and manuscript editor from Prentice-Hall, Doug Corcoran, the issue came up again in a round-about way. He was reciting to me a long and varied list of health topics that he hoped would someday be converted into publishable manuscripts. "Right now, I'm looking for a *really good* juice book," he mentioned with no real purpose in mind for doing so.

"Funny, you should say that, Doug," came the reply. "It just so happens that a few weeks ago at a convention I was at, there was this lady who came up to my booth and essentially asked me the same question." I then rehashed the matter for him in detail.

Thus, out of two totally unrelated incidents within weeks of each other, came this book. It is probably the most ambitious research and writing project I've ever undertaken in my 37-book career. After looking over a number of juice books which have already been published, I knew where my challenge lay. That was to create what the lady at the convention and my manuscript editor both wanted—*a really good* juice book!

If it seems I'm glad-handing myself right now, I'm not. I knew from the start that to do something like this, I had to be different and go where no other author of juice books had ever gone before.

First, there are 83 different juices covered in this book. (This includes the combined entries under BERRY and CITRUS JUICES and several twin juice blends such as DATE-FIG and GRAPE-RAISIN.) No other juice book in print comes anywhere near that number. I ought to know, because I took the time to count their respective entries just to make sure.

Secondly, none of the other juice books present the detailed information this one does on proper produce buying. Now you'll have a pretty good knowledge of what to look for when buying decent fruits and vegetables for your juicing pleasure.

Thirdly, the reader comes away from my book well-informed on the nutritional contents of virtually every juice presented. This enables him or her to correctly understand the particular vitamins and minerals inherent in every produce item juiced. That way, he or she will know which of several juices might be the best to drink for meeting certain nutritional deficiencies.

Fourthly, a large number of diverse anecdotes and case studies are given, which show specific advantages for individual juices. None of the other juice books utilize this kind of first-hand field experience as I do. With the exception of some occasional name changes where requested or necessary, all of the stories cited involve true-to-life situations in very real geographical settings. Even the bizarre ones, such as the guy swallowing broken light bulbs or the woman smelling men's armpits for a living actually happened just as I related.

The worth of any really good book, however, can be found in its layout. I've adopted here one of the key features that made my first *Heinerman's Encyclopedia of Fruits, Vegetables, and Herbs* (1985) such a smashing best-seller. That is to have not one but three separate indexes, for the most extensive cross-referencing you could ever hope to find in any health book. The table of contents offers an index of health problems with the appropriate juice remedies beside them and their particular page numbers. Then the general text is alphabetized for locating the juices in order of their appearance. Finally, there is a general index in the back for everything else not listed in the other two.

I've included at the end a special four-part Appendix, which covers other important aspects of juicing, such as which kind of juicer is the best for you; dynamic juice recipes which two professional juice therapists, a major juice manufacturer and myself helped to create; exciting ways for using leftover pulp if you own something other than a Vita-Mix; unique products and the names and locations of their manufacturers or suppliers; and last of all, a short list of other juice books for those desiring to expand their horizons on imaginative juice combinations.

Finally, after thinking I was finished with such an important work as this, I found myself going back through the manuscript a second time and adding many additional paragraphs after numerous health problems to describe *how* particular juices worked for each of them. These explanations don't appear in any other juice books to the extent they do here.

Now that the challenge has been successfully met and this wonderful and historic project is behind me, I've set my sights on yet two other goals. That is to write my third and fourth sequel in this *health encyclopedia* series—namely, *Heinerman's Encyclopedia of Berries, Nuts, Seeds, and Sprouts,* and *Heinerman's Encyclopedia of Spices, Flavorings, and Condiments.*

So I raise my glass of ugli fruit* juice and salute you, the reader, with a propitious toast: "Here's to great juicing adventure, happy guzzling, and good health! May the liquids in your life float away all your cares, sorrows, and problems."

—John Heinerman, Ph.D.
December 23, 1993
Salt Lake City, UT 84147

*NOTE: Ugli fruit is a type of citrus common to Jamaica.

CONTENTS

Part Two: Health Problems and Their Juice Solutions

TENDINITIS
THROMBOSIS
THRUSH
THYROID (UNDERACTIVE)
TICS
TONSILLITIS
TRAUMA
TRIGLYCERIDES ELEVATED
TUBERCULOSIS
TYPHOID

ULCERS
UPSET STOMACH
UREMIC POISONING
URINARY TRACT INFECTION

VARICOSE VEINS
VENOUS INSUFFICIENCY

VIRAL INFECTIONS

VISION (POOR)

VISION DISORDERS

VISION PROBLEMS

VITAMIN A DEFICIENCY

VOMITING

WEAK HEART

WHITLOWS

WHOOPING COUGH

WORMS

WOUNDS

WOUNDS AND SORES

WRINKLES

YEAST INFECTION

ALFALFA JUICE

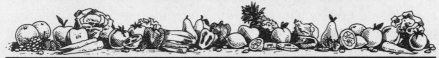

"Mineral Magic for Wounds and Sores"

DESCRIPTION

Alfalfa (*Medicago sativa*) for all appearances is a tall clover, with three-part leaves. The plant is a many stemmed and branched perennial, usually two to three feet tall when mature. The flowers are typically a lot like clovers, with the familiar purple, lavender, or blue tufts of blossoms interspersed at the ends of the stems. In fact, it is very difficult to differentiate between alfalfa and yellow and white sweet clover until they are actually in full bloom. Alfalfa is a very common plant in cultivation throughout much of the United States both for crop rotation, fodder, and medicinal herb purposes, but, as strange as it may seem, most people have never seen an alfalfa in bloom. It is a rather pretty sight to see!

NUTRITIONAL DATA

Without exception every standard medicinal herb book that I've looked through, written by famous or not-so-famous herbalists, invariably have made broad-sweeping generalities in regard to the presumed nutritional content of alfalfa. Yet not a single one of them has ever gone to the trouble of actually investigating the scientific literature in order to better understand the many different factors

1

governing this plant's nutritional contents. What I'm saying is that no other herb I know of shows so many fluctuations in its vitamin and particularly in its mineral contents as does alfalfa.

I refer more serious-minded readers to the excellent reference book, *Chemistry and Biochemistry of Herbage* by C. W. Butler and R. W. Bailey (London: Academic Press, 1973, Vols. 1-3). The many contributing editors show that the nutrient contents of alfalfa can vary drastically according to the moisture content of the soil, use of fertilizers, stages of maturity, any of the four seasons, temperature, rainfall, light intensity, length of stock grazing on it (if any), time of harvest, and so forth.

Suffice it to say, alfalfa is rich in vitamins A, C, K, and P, and these trace elements: nitrogen, phosphorus, potassium, calcium, magnesium, sulphur, sodium, chlorine, iron, copper, manganese, molybdenum, cobalt, zinc, iodine, selenium, chromium, vanadium, nickel, tin, and boron.

THERAPEUTIC BENEFITS

I'm reminded of a true story related by Henry G. Bieler, M.D. in his book, *Food is Your Best Medicine* (N.Y.: Random House, 1966, pp. 200-01) concerning alfalfa. Early in his career he happened to make a call in an unspecified part of rural Idaho. "I traveled across the sage brush for nearly a hundred miles to see a farmer who had suffered a discharging leg ulcer for several years," he wrote. "The whole right leg was greatly swollen and a foul crater was located just above the ankle."

Bieler knew that any type of alkaline vegetable juices would work, but it was late in the fall and there were no more garden vegetables available.

"Nor were there any supermarkets with daily supplies of fresh vegetables from distant farms," he added. In roaming outside to look for something green, he noticed the farmer's fields of alfalfa.

After announcing to the couple what he intended to give to his sick patient, the farmer's wife gave him a flabbergasted look. At first she thought he was joking, but soon realized he was earnest in his intention.

"I instructed her to gather the tender little alfalfa shoots, mince them very fine and mix them with water and grapefruit juice, which was available at a grocery many miles away." Besides this, the ailing fellow also was told to consume canned vegetables, whole wheat bread and raw cow's milk in the right proportions. "In time," Bieler concluded, "the ulcer healed entirely and the swelling disappeared. Needless to say, he never resumed his diet of hog fat, white flour and white sugar."

I frequently recommend fresh alfalfa shoots in combination with citrus or pineapple juices for any kind of open and runny infections which refuse to properly heal. I've even seen a few cases of gangrene in the early stages, completely reversed when alfalfa was consistently used.

Allergies.   Some nutritionally-minded doctors have reported in the medical literature a presumed connection between sugar intake and allergies. I myself noticed that whenever my intake of sweet things was up, my hay fever and allergy to a male cat named Jake, which I keep in my office, would be severe. Sugar produces an acid condition in the blood which alfalfa, however, can quickly turn around. The mineral salts in alfalfa will render the blood more alkaline. When this happens allergic reactions decrease dramatically. And when I monitor my sugar intake more closely, then the saliva on my cat's fur where he routinely licks himself clean, no longer bothers me as much.

Coronary Disease.   One of the causes of coronary disease is a buildup of fatty plaque on the walls of the heart arteries. Certain saponins within alfalfa leaves "scrubs" or removes this plaque away. Saponins are detergent-like compounds present in a number of meadow grasses, desert plants like yucca, and other herbs. If isolated and shaken up in a test-tube, they would manifest a sudsy appearance. It is this "soapy" property in alfalfa that, quite literally, "scrubs" away plaque by chemical action.

Gout.   Alfalfa is high in certain mineral salts, which actively promote kidney function. Several of these minerals are calcium, magnesium, and potassium. All of them are diuretic in nature and, therefore, help to remove fluid accumulations in muscle tissue and joints.

METHOD OF PREPARATION

Because the juice of fresh alfalfa leaves is much too potent to be
taken alone, it should be combined with grapefruit, pineapple, or
carrot juice to reduce the strong "boiled hay" taste and avoid possible
intestinal gas and unfavorable reaction by the liver. Remember here
that a *little* goes a long way!

Wash about two tablespoons of fresh leaves in a wire sieve. Set
your juicer (preferably a Vita-Mix for this recipe) on low speed,
somewhere between 1 and 3. Add the alfalfa leaves and one cup of
juice. Turn the switch on for about 15 to 20 seconds, then turn off.
Add another cup or two of juice, depending on how strong you like
your drink, and turn the machine on again for another 30 seconds.
The juice can be flavored with a pinch of cinnamon or cardamom,
if necessary, for an interesting but delightful "taste adventure."

APPLE JUICE

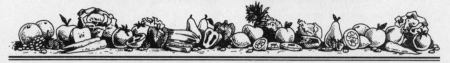

"An Apple a Day Keeps the Doctor Away"

DESCRIPTION

Botanically, apples (*Pyrus malus*) are members of the rose family and are related to pears and quince fruit. They are grown in the temperate latitudes of all continents. In North America, the northern half of the United States and the neighboring portions of Canada are apple country.

Apples are now available all year round. However, as late as the early 1900s, apples were not in season during the summer months. They were harvested in the fall and stored in cool areas. By late spring they were long in the tooth and would start to get soft and eventually rot. As better methods of refrigeration came into use, the apples were put in cold storage and had a longer shelf life.

While there are hundreds of documented varieties of apples, only about a dozen are grown commercially on a large scale. The top four varieties in the United States are the Red Delicious, Golden Delicious, McIntosh, and Rome Beauty, all of which are old standbys. (The Granny Smith, a newcomer, is rapidly gaining ground, however.) The Red Delicious accounts for more than 40 percent of the total tonnage of apples produced in America.

Though long on looks, Red Delicious falls a tad short on flavor. The golden delicious is similar in shape to the former, but is far juicier and sweeter and has a smoother flesh texture than red delicious does. When it comes to the taste test for apple juice, nine times out of ten the golden delicious will walk away with blue ribbon honors.

Apples

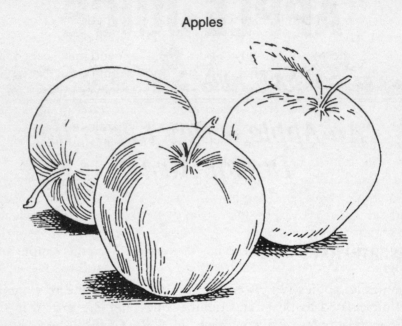

NUTRITIONAL DATA

One cup of apple juice contains 15 mg. calcium, 22 mg. phosphorus, 1.5 mg. iron, 2 mg. sodium, 250 mg. potassium, trace amounts of some B-complex vitamins, and 2 mg. vitamin C. An additional analysis commissioned by the Vita-Mix Corporation of Cleveland, Ohio shows the vitamin A content is 20 I.U. per 100 grams of apple juice and the presence of chromium was detected in 0.2 ppm (parts per million).

THERAPEUTIC BENEFITS

There are several things which make apple juice one of the most beneficial things for even the worst kind of constipation. First there is the high pectin content. Pectin is a water-soluble substance in many fruits and vegetables that yields a gel from which jellies are made. It is a natural cell scrubber derived chiefly from plant cell walls and fruit such as apples and different kinds of citrus. One apple yields about two grams of pectin. When it combines with certain mineral salts in an apple, they form an insoluble salt that has strong laxative properties.

If you think apple juice works fine for a plugged bowel, then you haven't seen anything until you combine it with one particular vegetable juice. The combination I'm about to recommend may seem a little revolting and not at all what your taste buds might be accustomed to but I'll let you in on a little "secret" of mine I've never put into any of my books before: when you combine *equal parts* of apple and *spinach* juice together, you have the most "dynamic duo" for cleansing, regenerating and reconstructing the entire intestinal tract!

I've put numerous clients on two cups of this apple-spinach juice per day for up to a week and have had testimony after testimony come back to me declaring how the most difficult cases of constipation, which *no* laxatives could begin to touch, had suddenly cleared up within a matter of days!

Just about everyone who has come away from this simple juice program with renewed health in their bowels, has asked me how it works so well. My response has been this: spinach is high in oxalic acid, which combines with the mineral salts and pectin in apples to form a unique substance with an incredible cleansing action to it. The closest thing that comes to mind to roughly illustrate how this works inside the bowels, is to compare it with the spray foam solution a housewife might put on the inside of her oven to get off all of the old, burned on matter which has collected there.

In a very similar way this remarkable substance formed from the combining of spinach and apple juice saturates the walls of the colon and, quite literally, through a strong but very safe chemical action "pulls off" old encrusted fecal matter that has accumulated over many weeks and months, if not years. Individuals who have been put on my simple combination juice therapy have reported actually feeling something working around inside of them. One woman described it as "a million little copper chore girls" (wire pot scrubbers) moving around inside. An older man, who had tried just about every prescription, over-the-counter, and herbal laxative on the market, exclaimed with glee when his regularity returned to normal once again, "It felt just like something was there inside of me stripping all the gunk off my colon walls!"

Additionally, consider setting some homemade apple juice aside in a glass container near a warm place for a week so it can gently ferment. You might want to give the jar a few good shakes during this period to agitate its contents even more. After this, you will have your own apple cider vinegar which can be taken in tablespoonfuls every day for arthritis. This is an old Vermont folk remedy made famous in the national best-selling book on apple cider vinegar written some years ago by a country doctor named Jarvis.

Arthritis.   One thing which his own observations had taught him was that when apple juice is *fermented*, it works better for arthritis than when it isn't fermented. Neither he nor other researchers who have studied the matter since then, know quite how it works. But the fact remains that measured doses ($\frac{1}{2}$ cup twice daily) of *fermented* apple juice, do indeed seem to help relieve arthritic pain. The way it does this is by reducing the acid crystal deposits which form around body joints.

Cholesterol and Triglycerides (Elevated).   Much has been said about cholesterol within the last decade; in fact, we've gone to an extreme in blaming cholesterol for many heart-related problems when the real culprit is triglycerides. The pectin in apple juice pulp has been studied for its effects in rabbits, monkeys, rats, and mice given large amounts of fat in their diets. Invariably, those test control animals receiving apple pectin showed remarkably reduced levels of cholesterol and triglycerides. But in order for it to be effective, the pulp must be included with the apple juice itself.

METHOD OF PREPARATION

When using apples for making juice, I recommend only those which have been organically grown. I do this not so much because of any sprays which might have been applied on them by growers, but simply because I believe they are higher in mineral content than those grown the conventional way. I also have noticed that Cortland, Granny Smith, McIntosh, and Golden Delicious are by far more active for treating constipation than other kinds of apples.

Select four apples and wash them thoroughly with soap and water if they're not organic. Then wash some spinach leaves under cold water and drain to get rid of excess liquid. Cut up enough leaves into three-inch squares to fill one measuring cup. Next wash one tied bunch of parsley.

Separately juice the apples, spinach, and parsley. There should be enough of each to yield one cup of apple and spinach juice and approximately one to two tablespoons of parsley juice.

Then add one cup of shaved or crushed ice to your Vita-Mix or food processor. Combine all three juices with the ice and blend at high 3 speed for one minute. Refrigerate until chilled, then drink one cup on an *empty* stomach every 4 hours.

You would be well advised to stay near a bathroom after consuming two cups within an 8-hour period!

APRICOT JUICE

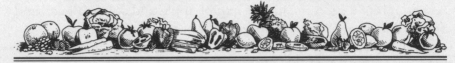

"Drinking the Fountain of Youth"

DESCRIPTION

Botanists have a bad habit sometimes of putting plants into categories where one does not expect to find them. Hence, they consider an apricot (*Prunus armeniaca*) to be a plum, and an Armenian one at that. In fact, this tree with fruit the color of brass or of old beaten copper originated in Central Asia a long time ago. It is still found growing in the wild between Bejing and the Great Wall of North China. The Romans and later the Arabs introduced it into southern Europe.

The tree yields lovely white blossoms when in full bloom. The ripe fruit has a sweet-sour taste to it. Different culinary experts have attributed the origin of the distinctive "sweet-sour" flavor so common to a number of Chinese dishes, to the use of the apricot. Now, however, it is merely sugar and vinegar that simulates the same thing.

NUTRITIONAL DATA

Apricots are incredibly rich in vitamin A, yield some potassium, and smaller amounts of phosphorus, calcium, vitamin C, and iron. The fruit also has a lot of sulphur in it, which accounts for the odd sourness.

10

THERAPEUTIC BENEFITS

Until a few decades ago, the Hunzukuts of Hunza Land were virtually unknown outside their extremely isolated valley in a land where six huge mountain ranges converge and the borders of China, Pakistan and the former Soviet Union meet. Just beyond the northern tip of Pakistan and nestled between rocky ramparts between twelve and twenty thousand feet high, lies a country where people never seem to get old.

Those who have had the rare privilege of visiting this health Shangri-La will know that the entire country is filled with tens of thousands of apricot trees yielding several million apricots annually. Yet, it is not often that even a single apricot goes to waste.

The apricots are split open, the stone removed and stored and the fruit left exposed to the sun and air to properly cure and dry; or they are either juiced, stewed, or baked. Even those which are bruised, damaged, or showing early signs of rot are put out to dry or used in some other way for food, cosmetic or medicinal purposes.

"Of all the things we have in this land," one village elder said, pointing to an orchard of apricot trees with a sweeping gesture of his right hand, "these alone are worth more to us than anything else you see around here!"

A wonderful oil derived from the apricot pits is used for cooking and to give the hair and skin richness and beauty. The pulp remaining after this oil has been extracted is fed to milking goats, cows, and sheep.

It is the innovative applications for which the juice is utilized, that I find the most exciting. In a land where electricity is virtually nonexistent and "invention becomes the mother of necessity," juice is obtained manually in different ways. It is used in place of water when making large flat pancakes called chappatis, often in place of milk over cooked oatmeal to give it an inspiring sweetness, and instead of water when cooking curried lamb and salted rice. A morning breakfast tonic will frequently be a shot of apricot juice, which makes a wonderful "wake up call" for the liver, pancreas, and adrenal glands to crank up the body's energy levels for the day.

Something else soon becomes apparent when a Western visitor starts roaming around inside this tiny kingdom. *Very few* of the older inhabitants have any wrinkles to speak of. To say that the majority of them are *virtually wrinkle-free* is not stretching the truth very far by any means.

When you stop to consider that these people are constantly exposed to the elements of wind, sun, heat, and cold 365 days of the year, and yet show *no* serious effects of such weathering in their skin, astonishment soon sets in. Now I'm pretty good at guessing people's ages because of my many years spent in the field as an anthropologist studying various cultures all over the world. However, you may find that when confronted with individuals who appear to be 30, 40 or 50, only to learn from them that they are *really* 50, 60 and 70, then your curiosity really sets in and the mind immediately goes to work trying to figure out the "beauty secret" at work here!

It's really no secret at all. It's just the apricots they consume so frequently in different forms with nearly every meal. Within apricots may be found those life-giving nutrients, such as vitamins, minerals, amino acids, enzymes, and oils that go to work to keep the skin fairly supple and young. Of course, the Hunzukuts have lifespans similar to our own, with just a handful reaching the century mark. However, the surprise in store for those who are able to go there is that they don't *look* old, even though they *are* old!

Cancer; Failing Eyesight; Second-Hand Smoke, Sluggish Liver.

All four of these health problems, while different in their clinical symptoms, nevertheless share a *common* factor. Each one of them positively responds to varying amounts of vitamin A. Apricots are high in what is called provitamin A or betacarotene. Their bronze color attests to that. Numerous studies reported in the medical literature of the last half decade point to vitamin A as being one of the very best chemopreventive and chemotherapeutic nutrients in coping with cancer. When the body is deficient in vitamin A certain vision problems occur. One is night blindness, which is an inability of the eyes to adjust to darkness. Another is xerosis, a disease in which the eyeball loses luster, then becomes dry and inflamed, thereby reducing visual acuity. A third is the development of sties in the eyes. But when vitamin A is continuously administered in such cases, they promptly disappear. Vitamin A therapy has also proved extremely useful in treating patients whose lungs have been continuously exposed to second-hand smoke. This nutrient protects the delicate epithelial tissues lining the respiratory tract and repairs any injury done to them by smoke, heavy metal contaminants, dust, or grain pollens. Next to the heart, the liver is the second most important organ in the body, performing several hundred different functions. If the liver can be likened to an NFL football team, then vitamin A is the star quarterback who see that his team is always winning and never defeated by sickness or injury.

METHOD OF PREPARATION

Wash and remove the pits from a dozen apricots. Put them in your blender and add one and one-half glasses (12 fl oz) of water. Blend together until thoroughly smooth, then drink and enjoy!

Another method which I've adapted from the Hunzas is to soak a package of dried apricots overnight in some bottled mineral water. Add honey and powdered cinnamon to taste before liquefying in a blender to a smooth consistency. For some variation, try adding one cup of refrigerated plain yogurt, or do the same thing with equal parts of soaked dried apricots and prunes for a really moving and healthy experience!

ARTICHOKE (JERUSALEM) JUICE

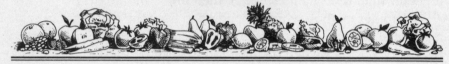

"A Dieter's Delight"

DESCRIPTION

The Jerusalem artichoke (*Helianthus tuberosus*), although an entirely different type of plant from the more familiar globe artichoke, resembles it in the flavor of the edible parts. It belongs to the sunflower family, having flowers with yellow ray petals, which make a fine show for a background or for a screen in the garden.

The plants grow to a height of six feet or better and have hairy leaves six to eight inches long. The stems usually are not branched. Jerusalem artichoke is a perennial and lives from year to year by means of its large tubers, which are edible and have a flavor somewhat resembling the globe artichoke. This probably explains the reason why it has been called "artichoke" rather than "potato," which its tubers greatly resemble.

There are a number of varieties differing especially in the color of the tubers. There are white, purple, red, and yellow-skinned varieties, but the flavor is not sufficiently different to be of much concern to the average consumer.

NUTRITIONAL DATA

One Jerusalem artichoke yields enough carbohydrate to equal one small baking spud. Most of this is a particular type of starch known as inulin, which is a form of fructose. Inulin (*not* insulin) is an efficient fuel for the body's energy needs. There is a fair amount of enzymes in the tuber as well.

THERAPEUTIC BENEFITS

Obesity is a national *disease* of epidemic proportions! So states the American Medical Association and allied health care associations. The inclination to eat often and the wrong kinds of food, besides lack of exercise and biochemical malfunctions, contribute to this widespread problem.

The key to understanding obesity is to know something about the taste buds located on either side of the tongue in your mouth. They transmit "flavor signals" to the brain of everything we chew and swallow. Those items which happen to be sweet and delicious, like chocolate, cream, or sugar, are bound to make a definite impression on the brain. In fact, such substances will be mentally isolated and held in a special place to be continually referred to.

At the same time this "preferred foods and beverages" file is being created, the brain is also producing certain biochemical "flavor markers" which circulate throughout the body in hopes of detecting *more* of such pleasurable substances. Upon not finding any, distress signals flash back to the brain which then commences creating biochemical cravings for these delicious things.

This is why many obese people constantly desire those foods which are sweet and tasty, but, unfortunately, are very fattening and unhealthy for the system.

The value of something like the Jerusalem artichoke, *when combined* with a small amount of carrot, alfalfa, or beet juice is that it tends to satisfy these cravings when consumed a certain way. Instead of being swallowed in the usual gulps, it is far better to *sip* this juice slowly through a straw. By doing so, the tongue has the added benefit of having the juice mixture run over its taste buds and linger a little longer inside the mouth before being swallowed. The brain becomes sufficiently appeased for awhile so that it cuts back on the amount of "flavor markers" it would ordinarily produce.

When this happens, the individual isn't faced with the mental or emotional temptation to snack. Willpower prevails and junk foods that add pounds to the body are simply not consumed. With moderate exercise, prudent eating habits, plenty of water (up to 6 full glasses a day), and the judicious use of culinary spices and herbs for setting the body's glandular "thermostat" a few degrees higher, stored fat—the most difficult thing to get rid of—can be biochemically "burned up."

The Jerusalem artichoke is just the thing to help accomplish this for those seeking a way to shed ugly fat *and keep it off for good!*

Chronic Fatigue Syndrome; Diabetes; Hypoglycemia. All three diseases share at least one major cause for their origins. Each one of them is related to blood sugar imbalances of some kind. In the case of diabetes, it is too much sugar and too little insulin to burn it up. But in the case of chronic fatigue syndrome and hypoglycemia, it's just the opposite: too little sugar in the circulating blood plasma and way too much insulin. This is a situation that is comparable to leaving the furnace on in July. The Jerusalem artichoke contains a starchy component called inulin. This is *not* related to what the pancreas produces, but is instead a unique carbohydrate which is quickly converted into an efficient energy that nutritionally supports those organs (liver, pancreas, spleen) responsible for normal blood sugar metabolism. Put another way, inulin stabilizes wildly erratic blood sugar levels. It does away with the yo-yo effects and maintains a blood sugar level somewhere in the center. Once this happens, these energy-draining problems are adequately corrected.

METHOD OF PREPARATION

Scrub and wash one Jerusalem artichoke tuber. Push through a centrifugal or masticating juicer with a wooden plunger. Mix that juice with an equal amount of carrot, alfalfa, or beet juice. Then slowly sip through a plastic straw, running the juice around inside of your mouth before swallowing.

ASPARAGUS JUICE

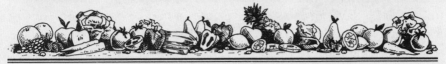

"Nourishing Tonic for the Kidneys"

DESCRIPTION

Asparagus (*Asparagus officinalis*) was grown as a food plant by European and Asiatic people long before the Christian Era began. It is now the common garden variety grown in just about every corner of the globe. It is a vigorous-growing bushy plant with finely divided or rudimentary leaves on long heavily branched stems. The stems die down every year, while the fleshy roots increase in size and number from year to year. A bed properly established in a garden can last a lifetime, if given the proper care.

There are about eight to ten different species of asparagus largely grown for ornamental purposes, but they have been used as sources of food by people living in the Mediterranean countries. Usually the tender sprouts are used, but in some cases the fleshy roots are used, and a few species produce a tuber which has been used. None of them, though, can compare with the present garden variety in yield, flavor or palatability.

NUTRITIONAL DATA

One cup of cut spears yields the following nutrients: 30 mg. calcium, 84 mg. phosphorus, 1.4 mg. iron, 3 mg. sodium, 375 mg. potassium,

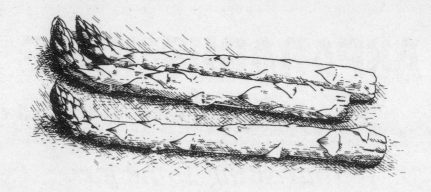

Asparagus

1,220 I.U. vitamin A, 2 mg. niacin, and 45 mg. vitamin C. In addition, asparagus contains several nutritionally significant trace elements: tin, molybdenum, and silicon. As the *Journal of Nutrition, Growth and Cancer* (1:183-196, 1983) reported "dietary tin has an affinity for the thymus," while the other nutrients are important for the pineal, adrenal, and thyroid glands as well as major organs such as the heart, liver, lungs, spleen, pancreas, and skin.

THERAPEUTIC BENEFITS

Maurice Mességué is one of Europe's greatest and most famous herbalists. Born in the remote French village in the Gers in Gascony, he learned at a very young age from his father the plant lore handed down by generations of his forebears: the special properties of everyday plants and flowers.

It was Mistinguett, the toast of Paris and the beloved of French film star Maurice Chevalier, who started him along the road to fame when he cured the rheumatism in her million-dollar legs. Through Mistinguett, Mességué encountered a whole new world he barely knew existed. He treated President Herriot of France, Ali Khan, King Farouk of Egypt, the Cardinal who eventually became Pope John XXIII of the Roman Catholic Church, and great artists like Maurice

Utrillo and Jean Cocteau. He became friends with Sir Winston Churchill, former British prime minister, and many other international celebrities.

He wrote several best-selling books detailing many of these healing experiences with herbs and included a number of his own remedies. They were *Des Hommes Et Des Plantes* (Paris, 1970) and *C'est La Nature Qui À Raison* (Paris, 1972), which became useful additions to my own ever-expanding library of books on medicinal plants and folk medicine.

One of the most remarkable cures mentioned by him involved the use of asparagus juice for treating a severe case of renal disorder. The patient was identified as one Gaston Valore, "a short, thick necked, heavyset man with a gluttonous appetite for any food his eyes set on."

The symptoms came on quite suddenly, about ten days after his patient suffered a sore throat. A rapid swelling of the face and legs was noticeable. Blood showed up in his urine. The man also complained of a migraine headache and severe pain in his groin. Mességué diagnosed the condition as acute nephritis or Bright's disease.

He took his patient off all of the rich foods and alcohol he had previously been consuming and put him on a very strict diet with little sodium and considerably reduced protein. He prescribed daily glasses of asparagus juice and as much water as his patient passed in urine the day before, plus one pint extra. He put the man to bed insisting that long periods of rest were absolutely essential to his recovery. Within 4-$\frac{1}{2}$ weeks the man was up and around, completely cured and enjoying life again, although at a more moderate and prudent pace.

Acne. This dermatological problem is often the result of poor diet. The average sufferer is usually a teenager or in his or her early twenties. Unfortunately the most popular foods are greasy and sugary. This results in an acid buildup in the blood. Because of its extremely high alkaline content, asparagus juice can reverse this condition in a very short time, if such foods are avoided. Once this happens, the skin begins to clear up because there are no more acid toxins to break through any more.

Eczema. This skin condition can be caused either by a nutrition-ally-deficient diet or mental and emotional stress. Both tend to create a lot of acid within the body. Since asparagus has a respectable amount of mineral salts, it can correct this condition very nicely, thereby making the blood more alkaline.

Skin Problems.   Quite a few skin ailments can be attributed to an excessive accumulation of acid within the system. When the body attempts to rid itself of such toxic waste materials, it will generally do so through the largest organ of elimination it has, namely the skin. But when asparagus juice is taken in sufficient quantities, it basically neutralizes all of this excess acid so it can be eliminated in other ways instead of through the skin.

METHOD OF PREPARATION

Buy the green variety which has more vitamins in it. Remove the tops and lightly steam them for a delicious side dish to any meal. Juice the tough stems in a centrifugal or mastication juicer in order to extract all of the rich mineral contents from them.

You'll soon discover that asparagus juice is quite alkaline on account of the mineral and trace element salts present. It also contains asparagine which enables the body to rid itself of toxic waste materials. In passing.through the system, it will impart an unusual odor to your urine. Don't be alarmed by this, as it only indicates that your body is being properly detoxified and your kidneys are functioning normally again.

Eight asparagus stems generally yield about one-half cup of juice. Because of its high alkalinity, you might want to dilute it in an equal amount of low-sodium vegetable or tomato juice. I wouldn't recommend something sweet like carrot juice; it's best to keep the alkalinity intact with another alkaline juice of some kind. Where the blood is extremely acidic due to the frequent consumption of meat, fat, sweet foods, soft drinks, colas and coffee, the use of asparagus juice will quickly turn this condition around and put the blood back into its usual healthy alkaline state.

AVOCADO JUICE

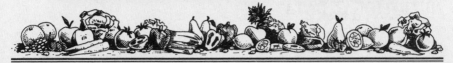

"Lubricating the Joints and Heart"

DESCRIPTION

Avocado (*Persea americana*) has an incredibly sensuous texture. Creamy with a delicate nutlike flavor, it can send the tongue into virtual ecstasy with its opulent and silky feel.

The tree from which it comes is related to the laurel and grows in a semitropical climate. Orchards extend from the California coastal city of Santa Barbara, down the Pacific side of the Western Hemisphere to Peru in South America. Each year, southern California alone harvests about 600 million avocados.

Believe it or not, the avocado is botanically considered to be a fruit, although it's more often used as a vegetable.

California avocados are available year-round. The Fuerte, a hearty variety that can withstand frost, is in stores from November through May. It is pear-shaped with smooth green skin. The pebble-skinned Hass, which originally took root voluntarily in the backyard of Rudolph Hass, is in season from April to November. Hass is more oval in shape with purple-black skin. Other varieties are also on the market, assuring us a constant, plentiful supply.

Avocados have the strange distinction of ripening only after they are picked from the tree. Most avocados are sold firm and must be softened before juicing or eating them. After purchasing some, let

21

them ripen in a warm, dry spot like the kitchen counter until they are soft, but not mushy, to the touch. At that point, if you are not ready to use them immediately, store in the refrigerator.

NUTRITIONAL DATA

One avocado contains the following essential nutrients: 23 mg. calcium, 95 mg. phosphorus, 1.4 mg. iron, 9 mg. sodium, 1,368 mg. potassium, 660 I.U. vitamin A, 8.6 mg. niacin, and 82 mg. vitamin C.

THERAPEUTIC BENEFITS

Throughout Central and South America the avocado is not only consumed with great relish, but also highly regarded for its extremely nourishing properties. It is a favored saying among the Maya Indians inhabiting the Yucatan Peninsula and the highlands of Guatemala that where avocados grow, "hunger (or malnutrition) has no friends."

Too many of us think only of avocados in the traditional Mexican sense of guacamole. But among the Mayan the avocado is considered to be a food which keeps the joints of the body moving freely and the skin young and supple. In fact, I've *never* once seen an older Mayan ever afflicted with rheumatism or arthritis so long as he or she regularly consumed ripe avocados in the diet.

Since one medium-sized California avocado contains about 300 calories, 88 percent of which are contributed as fat, it is little wonder that such a food can provide natural lubrication for the body's different joints—neck, elbows, wrists, hips, knees, and ankles.

Besides this, avocados used consistently in the diet can actually lower total cholesterol while maintaining high-density lipoproteins (HDL), or good cholesterol which protects against heart disease.

According to a study done by a group of Australian researchers and published in the *American Journal of Clinical Nutrition* (October 1992), a diet with between 20 percent and 35 percent of calories from the monounsaturated fat in avocados was actually better for reducing total cholesterol than a low-fat, high-complex carbohydrate diet.

The study undertaken at Wesley Hospital in Brisbane, solicited the services of 15 female volunteers, who all followed three different diets for three weeks each: their usual diet, a low-fat diet high in complex carbohydrates, and an avocado-enriched diet. With their usual diet, participants averaged 34 percent of their daily caloric intake from fat. On the carbohydrate diet, participants reduced fat intake to 21 percent by eating more breads, cereals, fruits, vegetables, and low-fat dairy products and by cutting back on margarine, butter, fatty meats and greasy snacks such as potato chips. On the avocado-enriched diet, which consisted of eating as well as *drinking* avocado meals, participants increased their overall fat intake to 37 percent by consuming about one avocado per day and by decreasing amounts of breads, cereals, fruits and vegetables.

Compared to the participants' original cholesterol levels, the avocado-enriched diet reduced total cholesterol by 8 percent, while the carbohydrate diet decreased it by 5 percent. The avocado diet maintained the HDL level, however, while the carbohydrate diet decreased HDL by 14 percent.

Various native tribes inhabiting those parts of Brazil, Colombia, Ecuador, and Peru that encompass the Northwest Amazon where wild avocados grow in abundance, are noticeably free of rheumatism, arthritis, and hardening of the arteries. Only when they become acculturated into the white man's dietary world and disregard their own traditional foods such as avocado, do they become obese, plagued with joint pain, and susceptible to coronary heart disease.

Dry Skin and Scalp.   Dryness of the skin and scalp may be due to environmental considerations, such as excessive exposure to sun, wind, and rain. These elements have a tendency to dry out the natural oils which the sebaceous glands routinely secrete. The extreme practice of avoiding all fats can also deny the body the necessary oil it needs for lubrication. Avocado is rich in oils and fats. In fact, I can think of nothing better which conforms to the "green herb for meat" idea conveyed by God unto Adam in Genesis 1:29 than this. When "Nature's own green butter" is regularly consumed, then the aforementioned glandulae sebaceae are able to secrete their usual oily semifluid sebum through the fine hairs covering that superficial thin layer of skin known as the dermis or corium. Internal glands similarly respond to the natural fat in avocado, enabling them to secrete their own fluids to keep our body muscles and joints limber at all times.

Malnutrition and Underweight. Both are pretty much synonymous with each other. Malnutrition can be due to poor assimilation, poor diet, or overeating. Usually though, it is often due to an inadequate diet, resulting in a dangerously thin physical appearance. By the time this critical stage has been reached, the body has pretty much utilized just about all of its stored fat resources. The only hope of reversing this is to slowly introduce more fat, which is readily digestible and can reduce this deficit. Avocado meets the necessary criteria for doing this.

METHOD OF PREPARATION

Peel a ripe avocado, making sure you do not cut into the flesh while doing so. You want to retain the outer membrane just beneath the skin, since this is where all the mineral goodness is located. This area is a slightly darker green than the rest of the inside flesh. After peeling, cut it in half and remove the inner pit.

Drop both halves into your blender. Add two cups of tomato juice and one level teaspoon of Kyo-Green and liquid Kyolic aged garlic extract (see Appendix). Then squeeze in a dash of lemon or lime juice. Season with a little granulated kelp. Set on variable low speed and mix for 1-½ minutes.

BANANA JUICE

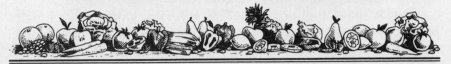

"Soothing the Suffering of Colitis and Ulcers"

DESCRIPTION

Bananas (*Musa sapientum*) are believed to have "originated some-where in Southeast Asia" and been "aboriginally introduced as far east as Hawaii" by ancient mariners from Panama or Colombia in the northern part of South America, ethnobotanist Paul Alan Cox claims in his book, *Islands, Plants, and Polynesians* (Portland: Dioscorides Press, 1991).

Regular bananas come in different lengths, from the small "finger" type to the larger kind we're used to. The yellow ones may be eaten raw, while the big green plantain bananas found in many semitropical regions of the world, must be cooked, steamed, boiled, baked or fried before being consumed.

All parts of a banana have some use in many indigenous cultures. Ripe fruits are peeled and sliced, dried and preserved, while green fruits are often scalded, peeled, sliced, sun dried, ground, and sifted to form a flour used for making mush and breads. Such flour keeps well and is good for treating a number of gastrointestinal problems (diarrhea, dysentery, and dyspepsia). The flower heads of many varieties are cooked and eaten in curries. The inner parts of the stem (called the cabbage) are eaten, diced, and boiled, or dried and made into a flour. Young shoots have served as vegetables.

25

Terminal buds of the inflorescences and immature fruits are sometimes used in curries. Young unopened buds in the center of the
stem are eaten raw or cooked. Rhizomes of certain varieties are
occasionally cooked and eaten. The unripe pulp of some types is
parched as a coffee substitute. The ashes of some of these plants are
used as a salt substitute sometimes.

I vividly recall during one of my several sojourns to the jungles
of Indonesia and Sumatra seeing a large piece of banana plantain
peel added to some wild monkey stew to take out the excess salt
and seeing some huge plantain leaves effectively employed as
temporary umbrellas and sunshades to protect inhabitants from the
monsoon rains and blistering heat. I'm reminded too of how the
unripe fruit of banana plantain has sometimes been pounded into
the hole of a bark canoe to plug up the leak; how the sap has been
used for snakebite or scorpion injuries; how the extract juice of the
leaf and bark has been used as wonderful antidotes for opium and
arsenic overdoses; and how the flowers have been used to treat
diabetes. I've also seen the ashes of a burned banana plant being
used by tribal witch doctors as an antacid for heartburn as well as
to staunch bleeding wounds.

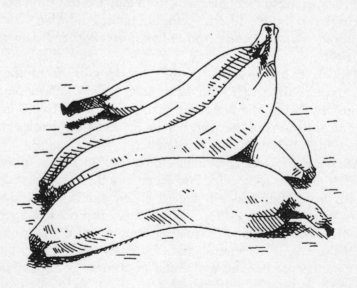

Bananas

NUTRITIONAL DATA

One large yellow banana contains the following nutrients: 11 mg. calcium, 35 mg. phosphorus, 1 mg. iron, 503 mg. potassium, 260 I.U. vitamin A, 1 mg. niacin, and 14 mg. vitamin C. A banana is also one of the few fruits to contain some trace amounts of chromium, a micronutrient responsible for stimulating enzyme activity in the metabolism of glucose for energy and the synthesis of fatty acids and cholesterol.

THERAPEUTIC BENEFITS

One of the most bizarre but highly effective uses I've ever heard for ripe bananas and banana juice was related to me recently by Jim Rose. Mr. Rose and the Circus Sideshow which bears his name, rolled into Salt Lake City Thursday, October 14, 1993, and performed the following Friday evening at a private lounge. His troupe had played at the same place and in the same month the previous year as well.

Mr. Rose was up to his usual act of shoving his face into broken glass, pushing ten-penny nails up his nose and ramming darts into his back. While being interviewed for a newspaper story before their show began, he shared with me something from their recent European tour. Recently Rose and his troupe gave several live radio and TV interviews in Amsterdam, Holland. Many interviewers "surprised" Rose by asking him to eat a light bulb on the air—and Rose felt he couldn't disappoint his fans by backing down. "I wound up eating five light bulbs in one day," he confessed, "and collapsed during intermission of that night's show."

Rose said he managed to recover by performing "lots of yoga exercises and eating and drinking the equivalent of nearly two dozen bananas or their juice" until the glass had completely passed through his system. "Those ripe bananas I kept juicing or pushing down me helped to heal my intestines, so I could continue performing," he stated. "Now I try to limit myself to *just one* light bulb a day, and I make sure I consume enough bananas afterwards," he concluded with a laugh.

Diverticulitis. Inflammation of the small pockets in the wall of the colon is something to take very seriously. They usually become filled with stagnant fecal material resulting in great pain. Fiber-rich foods can be quite irritating under such conditions. Because the flesh of a banana is soft and somewhat oily, it can be easily digested without posing any problem. By the time it reaches the colon, it has acquired enough mucus material to make it very slippery and slimy. In this state it coats the intestine walls and acts as an anti-inflammatory agent to promote healing.

Gastritis. When the mucosal tissue of the stomach becomes very tender and sore, the digestion of many foods can prove to be very difficult, if not excruciating. Banana juice coats, soothes, and relieves this serious inflammation much as the pink commercial antacid stuff frequently advertised on television.

Heartburn and Hiatal Hernia. The story of heartburn must focus on the lower end of the esophagus (foodpipe) just above the point where it leaves the chest by passing through the diaphragm to join the stomach. Normally the opening (called hiatus) through the diaphragm is tight enough to prevent the stomach from slipping up into the chest cavity. When that hiatus is too wide, a portion of the stomach may ride up into the chest; the anatomical result is described as a "hiatal hernia." This, in itself, need not be associated with heartburn. Rather, another structure—the lower esophageal sphincter (LES)—seems to be more important. The LES is that area of "muscular squeezing" by the wall of the lower esophagus that determines whether or not irritating stomach juices will back up into the esophagus. When the LES is too weak, backflow will occur. Now banana juice comes into play here to help solve both problems. First of all, it neutralizes the hydrochloric acid reflux felt in the back of the throat as a very unpleasant burning sensation. Secondly, it helps to "push" that portion of the stomach which has entered the chest cavity, back to its proper place. It neatly does this by creating a slippery condition to help the stomach slide back. So far as preventing heartburn goes, some of the minerals in banana, especially the potassium, strengthen the LES by promoting more even and frequent muscle contractions.

METHOD OF PREPARATION

There is one thing you should know about a banana: it is one tough item to juice! If you try juicing only one you'll end up with a creamy mush. I suggest adding 1–2 cups of pear, papaya, guava or mango juice along with a ripe banana in your blender.

Here's a delightful cocktail for your digestion that will heal even the worst case of intestinal inflammation. Into your Vita-Mix or blender put one half fresh banana (peeled), 1 cup mango juice, and 1 cup ice cubes. Turn on high speed for 15–20 seconds. The result is a very smooth, semi-sweet and extremely pleasant drink that will feel heavenly going down and is easy to digest.

BEAN SPROUT JUICE

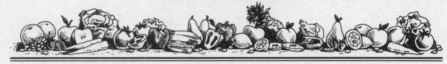

"Liquid Protein for Physical Stamina"

DESCRIPTION

The bean (*Phaseolus*) kingdom is one of the most varied in the plant world. Beans range in size from limas and kidneys, which are nearly an inch long, to pea beans, no more than $\frac{3}{8}''$ long. Almost every country has some traditional dish made with beans, and by the same token, these countries have their body of folklore about beans. Under most conditions, the bean is a prolific producer, and the inhabitants of South America and Southeast Asia still rely on beans as a staple item of their diet.

Most members of the bean family will sprout if viable beans can be found. Try beans from the supermarket, but be certain to remove beans that don't show evidence of sprouting. The advantage of sprouted beans is that they lose the gas-producing quality of unsprouted beans and become readily digestible. Each variety of bean sprout has its own distinctive taste. Beans that seem to sprout well include mung, navy, jack, kidney, pinto, fava, and lima.

30

NUTRITIONAL DATA

In the last couple of decades, sprouts have been "rediscovered" by nutritionists who have found them very rich in almost every important vitamin and mineral, while also containing adequate proteins to be classed as a "complete food." Many of the sprout proteins are predigested, for they are converted to amino acids during the sprouting process. The starches are also converted to simple sugars requiring little digestive breakdown, so they enter the bloodstream rapidly and are classified as a quick-energy food.

Sprouts also contain enzymes, the complex catalysts controlling many of the chemical reactions that take place in our bodies. We manufacture fewer and fewer enzymes as we age, and since foods cooked at temperatures greater than 140°F kill them, our stock of enzymes must be replenished by eating fresh produce. This is another reason for consuming home-grown sprouts.

The generous amounts of vitamin C contained in the tiny sprout is truly amazing. Many sprouts contain as much *or more* vitamin C as is found in an equal quantity of citrus fruit juices. Early investigations into the value of sprouts were conducted by Dr. Cyrus French during World War I. He selected troops suffering from scurvy and divided them into two groups. One group received four ounces of lemon juice a day, the others were given four ounces of sprouted beans. Within a month, over 70 percent of the bean eaters were free from scurvy symptoms, compared to just 53 percent of the lemon-juice takers.

As the beans begin to sprout, their vitamin content soars dramatically. The first early shoots of soybeans (per 100 grams of seed), for example, contained only 108 mg. of vitamin C in one study conducted at the University of Pennsylvania. However, after just three days, the vitamin C content shot up to 706 mg, an increase of nearly 700 percent! Similar comparisons can be made for other vitamins too, but the rate of vitamin increase during sprouting varies with each type of bean used.

I'm convinced, from all of the nutritional studies I've read over the years, that sprouts really do contain a varied and powerful battery of nutrients, rivaling citrus fruits in vitamin C and beef in protein, and surpassing almost any other known food source (except probably algae and seaweed) in completeness.

THERAPEUTIC BENEFITS

The best historical example of how marvelous a protein food bean sprouts are, is the Old Testament prophet Daniel. Ellen G. White, founder of the Seventh-Day Adventist religion said this about Daniel and his three friends in her *Counsels on Diet and Foods* (Takoma Park, Washington, D.C.: Review & Herald Publishing Association, 1938):

> "The youth [Daniel and his three friends]...were not only to be admitted to the royal palace, but it was provided that they should eat of the meat, and drink of the wine, which came from the king's table. In all this the king considered that he was not only bestowing great honor upon them, but securing for them the best physical and mental development that could be attained.

> "Daniel...decided to stand firmly [and] 'purposed in his heart' that he would not defile himself with the portion of the king's meat, nor with the wine which he drank.

> "Having by his courteous conduct obtained favor with Melzar, the officer in charge of the Hebrew youth, Daniel made a request that they might not eat...meat, or drink... wine. Melzar feared that should he comply with this request, he might incur the displeasure of the king, and thus endanger his own life. Like many at the present day, he thought that an abstemious diet would render these youth pale and sickly in appearance and deficient in muscular strength, while the luxurious food from the king's table would make them ruddy and beautiful, and would impart superior physical activity."

According to Daniel 1:11-12, he asked Melzar to bring him and his friends only "*pulse* to eat and water to drink" for the space of ten days. Then, he said, Melzar could judge for himself just who looked the ruddier in countenance, he and his friends on their simple diet or the other young prisoners dining on meat, wine, bread, and pastries from the king's table.

Several different Bible dictionaries have defined *pulse* as being "edible seeds and beans which are soaked and then eaten, as lentils, peas, beans, and the like," "which are eminently nourishing." See Samuel Fallows' *The Popular and Critical Bible Encyclopedia and Scriptural Dictionary* (Chicago: The Howard-Severance Co., 1907); and John S. Davis' *Davis Dictionary of the Bible* (Grand Rapids: Baker Book House, March 1978.)

The results were astonishing to Melzar. The 15th verse reads: "And at the end of ten days their countenances appeared fairer and fatter in flesh than all the children which did eat the portion of the king's meat." Or, as Ellen White noted:

> "Not only in personal appearance, but in physical activity and mental vigor, those who had been temperate in their habits exhibited a marked superiority over their companions who had indulged appetite."

Glandular Deficiencies.   Our bodies have many different glands which perform a variety of functions within us. These glands are dependent on various nutrients for proper nourishment. Amino acids are one group which help to accomplish this. Bean sprout juice contains many of the essential amino acids required for healthy glands.

Hormonal Imbalances.   A hormone is a chemical substance, formed in one organ or part of the body and then carried in the blood to another organ or part. Depending on the specificity of their effects, hormones can alter the functional activity, and sometimes even the very structure, of just a single organ or of various numbers of them. When an excess of one or several hormones results, the body's entire delicate mechanisms can be completely thrown out of kilter. Bean sprout juice can, in many instances, help to reduce an overproduction of certain key hormones, which, in their normal allotment are fine. This action on the part of bean sprouts may be attributed to their amino acids and enzymes.

METHOD OF PREPARATION

There is an assortment of qualified books to explain the intricacies of sprouting various kinds of beans and seeds. Only brief details can be given here. First, choose the beans to be sprouted. Second, measure out the amount you intend to sprout. Third, soak them in a quart pot of lukewarm water overnight. Fourth, pour the beans into your sprouter container the next morning, distributing them evenly over the bottom. Then thoroughly rinse them under cold water. Tilt the sprouter so that all excess water drains off. Set on top of the refrigerator or on the kitchen counter and cover with a damp hand towel or wet muslin cloth. Since sprouts grow best in the dark, be sure to keep them out of direct sunlight and artificial light as much as possible. Remember to rinse your seeds twice a day, morning and night, draining thoroughly each time you do this. By the 4th or 5th day your bean sprouts have matured enough that growth can be halted by refrigerating them.

To make a dynamic sprout drink, combine one cup each of apple juice and papaya syrup, one-half ripe, peeled banana, and three-fourth cup bean sprouts in your Vita-Mix or blender. Turn on medium speed for 50 seconds until a creamy consistency is reached. Chill and drink like a milk shake. A variation of this same recipe calls for equal amounts of pineapple juice and Perrier® water in place of the apple and papaya.

An incredibly nutritious soy sprout milk can be used as a substitute for real cow's milk for those individuals who are allergic to the latter. Blend one cup sprouted soybeans with four cups warm water and two tablespoons dark honey in your food blender for about five minutes. Then pour into a saucepan and cook over medium heat for about ten minutes, stirring constantly. Strain and allow to cool. Use the strained liquid as a delicious beverage over cereals, in making sauces and cream soups, and in any recipes calling for regular milk. Use the sieved residue as a filler in meat and vegetable dishes.

BEET JUICE

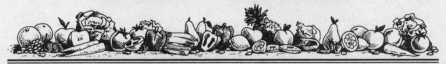

"Help Keep Yourself Cancer-Free"

DESCRIPTION

The common garden beet (*Beta vulgaris*) is probably a native of the Eastern Mediterranean countries, but is generally grown all over the world. It is very hardy and one of our more popular vegetable crops. It is an herbaceous plant that produces a fleshy root the first year and the seed stalk the second year.

There are three types of beets, but just one is agreeable enough to the digestive tract for human consumption. Stock beets or mangels are too coarse for human food but produce a tremendous amount of feed for chickens in the subsistence garden. Sugar beets, large and rather coarse in texture, contain 15 to 22 percent sugar and are the source of a large part of the sugar which we use on our tables. They can also be grown for chickens in smaller gardens.

Garden beets are a small, red type, probably developed by selection from the large stock beet. There are two general sub-types: the long, tapering, turnip-rooted type and the short or ball type. A flat type is usually classed with the ball type. They vary somewhat in inside color. The ideal color is a full dark red with no white stripes.

NUTRITIONAL DATA

Two whole beets contain the following nutrients: 14 mg. calcium, 23 mg. phosphorus, 0.5 mg. iron, 43 mg. sodium, 208 mg. potassium,

Beets

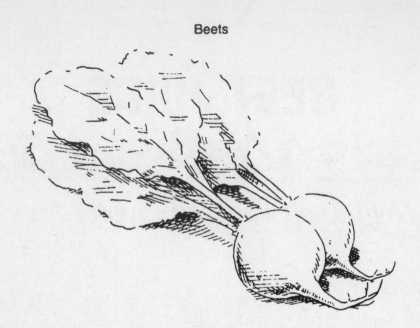

20 I.U. vitamin A, small amounts of some B - complex vitamins, and 6 mg. vitamin C.

The coloring principles present in red beet juice are known as betaines. These are a type of amino acids filled with ammonia. They consist mostly of betacyanins (red), with a small amount of betaxanthins (yellow). Betanin accounts for most of the betacyanins present. Plant chemists have discovered that this betanin occurs in red beet root as a sulphur-sugar complex.

A scientific quarterly that I edit recently published some original research conducted by a Hungarian physician, who found that beet root juice and its powdered form arrested the further development of many different kinds of cancer. The Spring 1993 issue of *Folk Medicine Journal* (1:98–104) reported on the work of Alexander Ferenczi, M.D. Working out of a district hospital in Csoma, Hungary, circa 1950-1960. Dr. Ferenczi observed with hundreds of cancer patients that raw, finely grated, powdered, or juiced beet root had remarkable chemotherapeutic properties to it. He hypothesized that "the very apparent red color may suggest that the active substance is the coloring matter."

Besides this, there is the hidden sulphur connection as well. Numerous studies conducted all over the world by doctors and scientists have demonstrated that fruits (figs), vegetables (cabbage, kale, kohlrabi, Brussels sprouts, cauliflower, mustard greens, watercress, radish), and certain spices (garlic, onion) which are rich in sulphur content, have a proven track record for preventing as well as treating tumors. Red beet root, as mentioned before, has small amounts of this very important trace element in various forms: the sulphur B-vitamins, biotin and thiamine; four sulphur amino acids, cysteine, cystine, taurine and methionine; and the sulphur-sugar complex known as betanin.

THERAPEUTIC BENEFITS

Dr. Ferenczi's original research (translated into English) is very exciting, to say the least, when it comes to the potent anti-tumor activity in beet juice. Test animals, which had been inoculated previously with malignant tumors and then permitted to drink beet juice at random, became virtually cancer-free and lived "on an average, 20 percent longer than the control animals" without the benefit of beets.

In administering it to many of his cancer patients, he soon discovered that while a number of the cancers went into remission, quite a few of them also got sick from the effects of the beet juice. He mentioned that their livers were unable to handle such large amounts of the concentrated juice. This unexpected side effect necessitated him to dilute the beet juice with water. Thereafter, no more unfavorable reactions occurred.

One case in particular serves to illustrate just how well beet root juice therapy worked for many of those whom he treated. A man aged 58 and only identified by the abbreviation D.J. was admitted to the district hospital in Csoma on January 5, 1956. He was suffering from an advanced lung tumor, probably due to excessive smoking. He had lost considerable body weight, had a high temperature, and a depressed immune system. He was put on diluted beet juice, grated beetroot salad, an iron supplement in tablet form, and hypodermic injections of neoperheparin and pyramidon. In two weeks, he filled out nicely, putting on substantial weight; his temperature returned to normal, and his immune system was running strong again. He was discharged and went home, but didn't stick with the regimen. A year later in late January, he returned to the hospital having suffered a serious relapse. Again beet juice therapy was employed in a valiant effort to save his life. For about two weeks it seemed as if he were making good progress, but suddenly his condition took a turn for the worse and he returned home in late May to soon die of lung cancer. Dr. Ferenczi pointed out that had the man faithfully stayed with the beet juice and not returned to his old habit of smoking, he would undoubtedly have lived for many years in a state of relatively good health.

Alcoholism. This physical dependence or addiction to alcohol is harmful to human health. It can lead to liver failure, dementia, pancreatic disease, and destruction of the heart muscle. There are only a few juices and herbs which can help restore these various organs to health again. Besides carrots, dandelion root, goldenseal root, ginko biloba, tomatoes, and turmeric, beet root juice is also very helpful. The organic mineral salts in these items rebuild tissue cells severely damaged by prolonged exposure to alcohol.

Drug Addiction. Drug abuse is pervasive in our society. It may be defined as the improper use of any drug, including: (1) Drugs legally prescribed and then used improperly by a patient; (2) legal drugs obtained illegally and used without a doctor's prescription; (3) illegal drugs. The addiction problem crosses ethnic, gender, and age boundaries: black, white, and brown, male and female, from elementary school to senior citizen. Organs most adversely affected are the brain, heart, lungs, liver, and kidneys. Because beet root is basically a blood-building herb, it detoxifies the blood and then renews it with minerals and natural sugars. Thus reconstituted, the blood can bring important nourishment to each of the aforementioned organs that have been greatly weakened by drugs.

Venous Insufficiency. This condition is common in older people, where there is often an inadequate drainage of blood in the veins from a particular place in the body. The result is usually an accumulation of an excessive amount of watery fluid in muscle tissue or the appearance of single or multiple skin lesions somewhere on the body. But the mineral salts and carbohydrates in beet root can increase circulation to such areas of the body and get the stagnant blood quickly removed.

METHOD OF PREPARATION

Juice one small beet in either a centrifugal or mastication juicer. Then in a food blender or Vita-Mix, add this juice or its equivalent organic beet root juice powder, 2 tablespoons (see Appendix), along with ½ bunch parsley, 3 leaves Romaine lettuce, 3 small carrots, one tablespoon of Kyo-Green chlorophyll powder, and one teaspoonful liquid Kyolic garlic extract (see Appendix). Set on a medium variable speed and thoroughly blend for about one minute.

This makes one of the best tonic drinks for the liver that I've ever tasted. It is excellent not only for cancer sufferers, but also quite useful in the prevention of that disease as well. Recommended intake for cancer is one glass each day; otherwise, one or two glasses weekly is sufficient for preventive measures.

Beet juice is one of the very best tonic drinks for the liver. However, *raw* beet juice, as Dr. Ferenczi himself discovered, can be extremely potent and cause the body to react in an unfavorable way when too much is taken at once. I once spoke with Ann Wigmore, the octogenarian founder of the Hippocrates Health Institute in Boston, about this very thing, and she recommended that raw beet juice should be mixed with some other kind of vegetable juice such as carrot or mixed greens to dilute its potency somewhat. I've discovered that *powdered* beet juice concentrate, when reconstituted (one tablespoonful to an 8 oz glass of water) can be taken alone on a daily basis without any unpleasant side effects.

BERRY JUICES

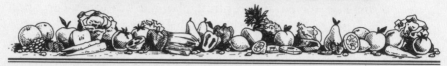

"Nature's Tasty Medicine"

DESCRIPTION

Berries of different descriptions are botanically classified as a type of fleshy fruit. True berries such as blueberry and tomato which is a fruit and not a vegetable (believe it or not), have many seeds in them. On the other hand, aggregate fruit, which has many small drupelike parts united into one structure (blackberry and raspberry), are popularly called berries but, in fact, really don't qualify as such.

With the advent of warm weather comes the introduction of all types of berries. They come in a wide range of shapes, sizes, and colors and grow in such contrasting environments that they can be found just about anywhere you go in the world. Berries not only taste good, but they also have wonderful medicinal properties to them as well. They may be summed up as cleansers, disinfectants, eliminators, and soothers.

Berries are at their best plump and fresh off the bush or tree, but many medicinal formulas and cooking recipes call for the juice. Their real benefits lie in this form. You don't need a juicing machine for berries since the juice is so easily extracted.

The simplest and perhaps oldest method of juicing is pouring hot water over crushed berries, letting them sit for an hour, then straining off the juice. They may also be placed in a jar of water under the hot summer sun for a day, then strained. The water dilutes the juice, but even when modern juicers and strainers are employed, it's still best to add water to the pure juice before drinking because the sugars are so concentrated.

Berry juice has a refrigerant property to it. This means that in time of fever, sunstroke, or to quench thirst in the heat of a hot summer day, nothing cools the body down as effectively as berries do. In fact, berry juice of any kind is remarkable for its ability to readjust the body's own internal thermostat to a more comfortable and healthier setting.

The following ten berries represent the most popular types with food, beverage, medicinal, or cosmetic appeal to them.

Blackberry (*Rubus villosus*). This is a shiny black fruit that grows on bushes that are so thorny they are called bramble. Even so, the taste of these sweet-tart berries lures country folk back to the bramble bushes during the summer months. They are the late summer and early autumn cousins of raspberries. They are also among the most perishable of berries, lasting just a few days in the refrigerator after harvesting. Other lesser known but equally delicious blackberry relatives are the loganberry and tayberry. Both are blackberry-raspberry hybrids. The juicy dark red boysenberry is a cross between the blackberry and loganberry. The sweet black olallie and the marionberry are much-prized trailing blackberries.

Black and Red Currant (*Ribes nigrum, Ribes rubrum*). These small black or red berries are rather tart for eating raw. They are closely related to gooseberries. Both kinds, as well as a white variety, are more popular in Europe than in North America. They appear from early to mid July.

Blueberry (*Vaccinium gaylussacia, Vaccinium corymbosum*). This is a familiar fruit with a deep blue skin and a whitish bloom. It goes by different common names, depending on which part of the country you're in: hurtleberries, bilberries, or whortleberries. There are two major types of blueberries: the low bush and the high bush varieties. The low bush has very small berries of a good flavor. The high bush berry is much bigger, tastier, and juicier, and the one we usually buy fresh in supermarkets or from farmers' markets. Its peak season is from June to August.

Boysenberry (*Rubus ursinus* var. *loganobaccus*).   Rudolph Boysen, an American horticulturist of the 1920s wondered what would happen if he genetically crossed several blackberries and raspberries. The result was a type of very large, juicy, delicious, aromatic berry that often reaches two inches in length. Boysenberries are thornless for easy picking and almost seedless. When fully ripe, they're deep, rich maroon—almost black in color—and ooze with juice. They ripen over a two–month period beginning in early June and thrive in southern and Pacific Coast areas where the winters are relatively mild. They have a distinctive raspberry flavor.

Cranberry (*Vaccinium macrocarpon*).   The Wampanoag Indians welcomed the Pilgrims of Plymouth Rock fame with berries they called *ibimi*, or "bitter fruit." But the Pilgrims, who thought the vines' long, pink blossoms resembled the heads of cranes, dubbed the crunchy, red berries "crane berries." Today, cranberries are enjoyed worldwide, but the story of their cultivation remains intricately linked with the history of Plymouth County, Massachusetts, where half the national crop is still grown. The cranberry is one of three fruits native to America (Concord grapes and blueberries are the others). For years, the early colonists harvested the fruit from wild-growing vines. In 1816, Cape Codder Henry Hall discovered that the berries grew especially large and juicy in the acid-peat soil found near sand dunes at the beach. Realizing that it was the combination of acidity and sand that made the difference, he planted more vines near the dunes, and thereby sparked such a frenzy for cranberry growing that the berries became known as "red gold." It takes from three to five years for a plant to mature, but once the vines blossom, they will bear fruit almost indefinitely.

Elderberry (*Sambucus canadensis, Sambucus nigrum, Sambucus racemosa*).   The elder shrub can grow from one to ten feet, mostly in width. It spreads underground and eventually forms thickets, sending up many young stems from the roots. Elder is scarcely woody, having a large white pith. The leaves consist of an average of seven leaflets which are pointed at the tips, toothed, smooth, or more often hairy beneath. Elder flowers are white and usually gather on just a few of the stems as a rule. The berries are of different colors, being more commonly purple and black, and very rarely red, green, or yellow. After they begin maturing in August, they measure about a quarter-inch in diameter and are juicy.

Gooseberry (*Ribes grossularia*).   Gooseberry and currant both belong to the same *Ribes* family of fruits, whose characteristics include thin translucent skins with soft, tiny-seeded fruit inside. This class of fruits, which have wonderfully pungent, tart flavors, are far more readily available in Europe than in the United States, although that is beginning to change. Gooseberry has been described as looking a lot like a "little green basketball with a stem on top," because its skin has striated lines which appear to divide the fruit into uneven sections. The sweet varieties are eaten fresh by some people; the more sour varieties make excellent preserves or are used in many desserts. However, most Americans seem to find the berries pretty sour, even when dead-ripe.

Huckleberry (*Vaccinium myrtillus*).   This is the wild blueberry namesake for Tom Sawyer's boyhood friend, H. Finn, who took to sailing the mighty Mississippi river on a raft. The fruits are blue and often confused with blueberries, but they are smaller. Whereas the only evidence of the blueberry's seeds may be in your teeth, the huckleberry has ten to twelve fairly large seeds. Huckleberry's flavor is more delicate than the blueberry.

Red and Black Raspberry (*Rubus idaesus*, *Rubus crataegifolius*, *Rubus occidentalis*).   In appearance, the black raspberry bears resemblance to the red, yet its color is darker and its shape tends more toward that of a "skull cap" than the "ball shape" of the red raspberry. The black species is a very seedy berry, whereas its red counterpart is less seedy and more juicy. The season for both begins mid- or late June and extends for only about four weeks.

Strawberry (*Fragaria ananassa*).   The leaves and flowers grow on petioles and stalks directly from the rootstock, which also produces long, rooting runners. The thin, light green leaves are divided into three more or less ovate, coarsely toothed leaflets and are lightly hairy on the lower side, at least on the veins. The small white flowers grow in raceme-like clusters during May and June. The familiar red "berry" is actually the enlarged, fleshy receptacle (the flower-bearing tip of the stalk), which holds the seedlike fruits on its surface. This fruit is native to America, available year round, with peak supplies available from April to June. It is enjoyed in other parts of the world, too.

NUTRITIONAL DATA

Berries contain a naturally occurring plant phenol known as ellagic acid. Scientists have observed that indigenous people who subsist on a lot of berries and nuts are virtually free of cancer. Although researchers have yet to actually define the exact mechanism of this cancer inhibition, they suspect that the ellagic acid found in berries and other natural foods, competes for DNA receptors that are also used by chemically-induced carcinogens. Two groups of mice received bi-weekly applications to their skin of a polycyclic aromatic hydrocarbon (PAH) carcinogen for four months. Compared to controls, mice pretreated with ellagic acid from berries had 45 percent fewer tumors per mouse and the latent period before tumor appearance was prolonged from six to ten weeks. This study, which appeared in the May 1986 issue of *Cancer Research* (46:2262-65), suggested that the inclusion into the diet of ellagic acid-rich foods like nuts and berries could significantly reduce the risk of cancer development by environmental chemicals.

Berries To The Rescue.   Berries tend to be rather high in potassium. Potassium is a mineral critical to the success of controlling high blood pressure. Potassium also helps to restore normal function to the kidneys, where the symptoms of hypertension begin. Therefore, berry juice of any kind will always be good in treating kidney and blood pressure related problems.

Berries are also rich in iron. Iron is important for the production of red blood cells within the body. Women seem to need more iron than men do; therefore, berry juices should be a routine part of their diets.

Berries also contain measurable amounts of vitamins A and C, and calcium and phosphorus. Both vitamins are necessary for supporting strong immune defenses, while the two minerals keep bones and teeth firm, and the heart and skin healthy.

Where berries really shine nutritionally is in their remarkable trace element contents. While not exactly equal to better known sources for such micronutrients as seafood, seaweeds, and algae, berries are one of the very few plant foods (along with some nuts and seeds) that contain a sufficient variety of trace elements to benefit the body.

Trace elements are vital for a number of different bodily functions. However, they seem to be especially important when it comes to certain glandular (pineal, thyroid, thymus, adrenal) and organ (heart, liver, stomach, pancreas, spleen, kidney, brain) operations.

Over a decade ago, the trace element composition of a number of berries was published in a report prepared by food chemists at the University of Helsinki in Finland for the scientific journal *Acta Agriculturae Scandinavica* (Supplement 22:89-113, 1980). The berries mentioned included: bilberry (huckleberry), lingonberry, cranberry, cloudberry, strawberry, black and red currant, gooseberry, rosehip, rowanberry, and raspberry.

While the researchers noticed that "wild berries showed exceptionally high levels of manganese, about ten times as high as cultivated berries and fruits," both types had appreciable amounts of a number of important trace elements. It is not possible to list the minerals for every berry here, but I've chosen red and black currants as composition models of what is fairly typical for the other berries.

The table below shows the content range for a number of trace elements occurring in both species of currants.

MINERAL	RED AND BLACK CURRANT	
Potassium	3.1-3.4 grams	
Calcium	0.40-0.72 grams	
Magnesium	0.14-0.24 grams	
Phosphorus	0.47-0.58 grams	
Sulphur	0.16-0.23 grams	
Iron	7.9-12 milligrams	
Copper	5.4-19 milligrams	
Manganese	1.9-3.1 milligrams	
Zinc	2.0-3.1 milligrams	
Molybdenum	1.6-3.8 milligrams	
Cobalt	5 micrograms	*(continued)*

MINERAL	RED AND BLACK CURRANT
Nickel	0.05-0.1 milligrams
Chromium	10-50 micrograms
Fluoride	0.1-0.2 milligrams
Selenium	1-2 micrograms
Silicon	10-50 milligrams
Rubidium	2.4-3.2 milligrams
Aluminum	3-16 milligrams
Boron	1.8-2.1 milligrams
Bromine	1 milligram

The trace element composition in other types of berries either comes close to or sometimes even exceeds these figures. Strawberries, for instance, have 1.4-2.3 grams potassium, 4.3 milligrams manganese, 4-10 micrograms cobalt, 2 micrograms selenium, 20 milligrams silicon, 3-8 milligrams aluminum, and 1.7-2.1 milligrams boron.

THERAPEUTIC BENEFITS

Blackberry. Herbert Langford, M.D., a professor at the University of Mississippi in Jackson, recommends the consumption of blackberries or their juice for treating hypertension. His research has shown that the high amount of potassium in the juice will help to bring down elevated blood pressure. Winona Rider, a Registered Nurse from Montgomery, Alabama finds that blackberry juice helps people suffering from anemia and that it also lessens the flow of excessive menstruation in some women. Some blackberry juice heated on the stove and slowly sipped through a plastic straw while very warm is good for alleviating the worst kind of cough, she insists. Blackberry juice is also good in the treatment of rheumatism, tonsillitis, heart problems, diarrhea, chronic appendicitis, acid indigestion, colitis, gallstones, and some hernias.

Black and Red Currant. Black currant is rich in vitamin C and the bioflavonoid rutin, which makes the juice very good to use for minimizing bruising, bleeding gums, slow leakage of the tiny blood capillaries, hemorrhoids, and connective tissue problems. Black currant juice also contains a small amount of gamma linolenic acid or GLA, while the whole berries have even more in them. GLA is vital to health because it helps the body to produce an essential hormone-like substance called prostaglandin PGE-1, which controls every organ in the body and which keeps the immune defenses strong. This particular prostaglandin and others like it, serve as biological regulators, controlling the action of the body cells and organs. They have a very short life of about one second and are only produced by the body when and where they are needed, each one having a unique and specific effect. Without the GLA from blackberries and their juice, not enough of these important prostaglandins would be produced. Blackberry GLA is also essential for the muscle locomotion and nerve transmission; in diseases such as multiple sclerosis it is of considerable benefit.

Red currant juice is wonderfully antiseptic and good for liver jaundice, ptomaine poisoning, and too much acid in the bloodstream. A story is told by one British herbalist, Mary Thorne Quelch, of a man in Liverpool, England consuming an entire pheasant at a holiday celebration and then being rushed to the local hospital soon thereafter suffering from ptomaine poisoning. The physicians on duty were able to save his life, but accredited it more to their patient having consumed a lot of red currant jelly, which had been served as part of the "trimmings" of the meal he ate. Both black and red currant juice are ideal for yeast infection in the mouth (thrush) or vagina (vaginitis). When served hot, they will induce perspiration and help to break up a cold or fever in much the same way that heated lemonade does.

Blueberry.   The juice is good for gout, kidney stones, chronic diarrhea, dysentery, sore throat, leucorrhea, typhoid, eczema, psoriasis, and rash. Medical researchers in Israel recently discovered that blueberries and their juice have bacteria-fighting properties which work against urinary tract infections (UTIs) in much the same way that cranberry juice does. Dr. Nathan Sharon, a biochemist at the Weizmann Institute of Science and Tel Aviv University, found that the juice contains a compound that weakens *Escherichia coli*, the chief cause of UTI, by preventing the bacteria from clinging to the cells along urinary and digestive tract linings. Sharon believes that drinking the juice of blueberry or cranberry is more of a preventive measure against UTIs than an actual treatment.

If you want to preserve blueberries without having to freeze them, try salting them. I learned this trick from an old French Canadian trapper up in the Northwest Territories, who lived in a region so remote that "even the geese need a compass to find out where they're flying," he joked. Here's how he told me to do it: Check the blueberries over, putting aside any broken, bruised, or overripe juicy ones for immediate use. Put the firm ones, dry into quart bottles leaving about one inch of head room. Colored glass should be used unless the berries can be stored in a completely dark area. Once they are in the bottle, add one teaspoon of ordinary table salt and agitate gently. Seal it; a screw-top bottle, hand tightened, is adequate. Without further shaking, put it into storage in any available, preferably dark spot. They will keep *almost indefinitely*! The berries will create a small amount of juice but remain firm. They neither ferment nor spoil. If the room temperature alternates somewhat between warm and freezing, be sure to let the bottles cool outside a few minutes before opening them, or just unscrew the lid very carefully by holding a cloth over it until you hear the hiss of air. If these simple precautions are not taken, and a bottle is opened immediately, the contents will, quite literally, explode all over you, the ceiling, and the walls. Take my word for it!

Boysenberry. Swirling a little bit of boysenberry juice around in the mouth and running it over the gums with your tongue, will prevent gingivitis, cold sores, pyorrhea, and bad breath. So claims a retired dentist I know from Lexington, Kentucky, who used it often enough in his practice and recommended it to most of his patients. Boysenberry juice will help to prevent scurvy, that dread nutritional deficiency disease that wreaks havoc upon the skin and nervous system. Boysenberry juice also makes a gentle laxative for older people, who are occasionally constipated and who require something moderate to promote an easy bowel movement. Boy-senberry juice is also excellent for alcoholics who want to quit, but need a comparable substitute to stave off the craving for more liquor. For this addiction, it is best sipped slowly through a plastic straw, and swished around in the mouth before swallowing, instead of gulping it down directly. By doing so, the taste buds along either side of the tongue send signals of pleasure to the brain, which then becomes satisfied enough to shut off the strong craving instincts for awhile.

Cranberry. Cranberry juice is very good medicine for the urinary tract. Lieutenant Commander Peter Sternlieb, M.D., formerly with the U.S. Naval Hospital in St. Albans, New York, used this often as an effective remedy in treating many cases of kidney infection and stones. His letter, which appeared in the January 3, 1936 *New England Journal of Medicine* (268:57) explained his therapy this way:

> "It has been my experience that the administration of cranberry juice is efficacious in conditions in which urinary acidification is indicated. Quinic and benzoic acids in cranberries are presumably the precursors of the hippuric acid that is excreted by the kidneys and thereby acidifies the urine...
>
> "The usual dosage of cranberry juice varies from 12 to 32 ounces daily. Simple pH determination of the urine can serve as a guide for effective dosage. I have found that an 8-ounce glass of cranberry juice four times daily for several days followed by 1 such glassful twice daily is a valuable adjunctive therapy and prophylaxis in stone-forming patients whose renal stones are more soluble in an acid milieu and in patients with certain urinary-tract infections."

Cranberry juice may also be good for an underactive thyroid. Iodine is a beneficial trace element for this particular gland, but ordinarily it's only found in seafood and sea vegetation such as kelp, dulse, bladderwrack, and shrimp. However, because of the nearness of the sea to many of the Massachusetts bogs in which cranberries are grown, their iodine content has been reported as being 35 parts per billion, according to the *Journal of Biological Chemistry* (79:409-11, 1928). Murdock Pharmaceuticals makes a Cranberry U.T. powder in gelatin capsule form, which some naturopathic and homeopathic doctors and chiropractors have used with success in treating urinary tract infection. This is a useful alternative to the juice for those with blood sugar problems who can't handle too many sweet things. (Murdock Pharmaceuticals is a division of Nature's Way Herb Co. in Springville, Utah.)

Elderberry. The juice is good for swollen tonsils and internal swelling of different glands such as the lymph nodes. It is particularly useful to give to children suffering from measles, mumps, and chickenpox. It helps to reduce fevers and eases earache when a few drops of the very warm juice are put into the ear canal with an eye-dropper. As a wash for the skin, the juice is unsurpassed in dealing with eczema, psoriasis, and poison ivy/oak rash. For cases of open or running sores on the legs, mix equal parts of brandy and elderberry juice and wash the afflicted areas twice daily. Bathing the skin with the juice in cases of erysipelas and lupus erythematosus is highly recommended. And in cases of burns and scalds to the skin, poultices of cold elderberry juice work wonders! It is also very useful in the treatment of gout. Most of the uses mentioned here in connection with elderberry juice originally came from remedies once employed by different Native American tribes residing in the eastern United States and upper Canada in the 18th and 19th centuries.

Gooseberry.   The juice is very good for any type of liver dysfunction that leads to a sudden onset of such symptoms as anorexia, coated tongue, constipation, headache, dizziness, pasty complexion, and, rarely, slight jaundice. The juice makes a wonderful lotion for erysipelas, St. Anthony's fire, Rosenbach's disease, and similar disorders which are marked by an acute skin inflammation and sharply defined with numerous eruptions. A combination of elderberry and gooseberry juice make an ideal lotion or wash for such conditions.

Huckleberry.   Dr. Elizabeth Barrett-Connor of the University of California at San Diego and Dr. Kay-Tee Khaw of Cambridge University in England published a study in the January 29, 1987 edition of *The New England Journal of Medicine* in which they stated that the risks of stroke could be reduced by nearly one half by increasing the body's supply of potassium. They pointed to fresh fruit, especially berries, huckleberry in particular, for helping to control the nation's third leading cause of death, after heart attack and cancer. One glass of huckleberry juice twice a week is sufficient for this protection. Huckleberry juice is also useful for typhoid, malarial, rheumatic and scarlet fevers. It makes a dandy lotion for eczema and psoriasis. One of its more recent uses has been found in the field of ophthalmology. French, Italian, and German medical researchers have published clinical studies showing that huckleberry juice exerts a positive effect in the treatment of capillary fragility, blood purpuras, cerebrovascular disturbances, venous insufficiency, varicose veins, dysmenorrhea, and microscopic hematuria caused by diffused and kidney capillary fragility. However, the prime application of the remarkable anthocyanosides in huckleberries and their juice has been in vision problems such as retinitis pigmentosa, poor night vision (nyctalopia) or its opposite counterpart, day blindness (hemeralopia), cataracts, diabetic-induced glaucoma, and myopia. The anthocyanosides in huckleberry have a definite affinity for the pigmented epithelium or retinal purple of the retina which composes the optical or functional part of the retina. Their effect on collagen structures in the eye explains the role in the prevention and treatment of glaucoma. The huckleberry juice compounds may also offer significant protection against the development of retinal (macular) degeneration and cataracts, particularly diabetic retinopathy and cataracts. Such huckleberry compound extracts are being widely used throughout Europe in the prevention of diabetic retinopathy. All of this work with huckleberry in ophthalmology actually began back in World War II when some Royal Air Force pilots in Great Britain swore that eating huckleberry jam or drinking huckleberry cordials prior to flying night missions over Germany significantly improved their visual acuity in the darkness. Such reports generated a lot of interest in the medical community in Europe, which led to a number of studies being done with the berry.

Red and Black Raspberry. The juice from both species of raspberry is wonderful for the following health complaints: anemia, hypoglcyemia, hypertension, labor pains during pregnancy, morning or motion sickness, fatigue, common cold, influenza, scurvy, stomach ulcers, heart problems, kidney stones, fever, painful menstruation, diarrhea, yeast infection, sexually transmissible diseases and poor circulation.

Strawberry. The juice is good for weak vision and blood-shot eyes when taken internally. The *Journal of Food Science* (41:1013, 1976) reported that poliovirus was inactivated with strawberry juice extract; it also inactivated the herpes simplex virus as well. Brushing the teeth occasionally with *thick* strawberry juice will prevent tartar buildup and gingivitis. If equal parts of strawberry and raspberry juice are taken once or twice a week, it will help to eliminate toxic accumulations in the circulating blood plasma; this is good for acne, blackheads, boils, carbuncles, and rough, unhealthy skin.

Bruising.   A bruise is caused by bleeding into the skin. Most bruises are due to injuries that damage the tiny blood capillaries just under the skin but do not actually cut or break the skin. Bruising may be caused by any one or several of the following problems: allergic reactions, anemia, Cushing's syndrome, adverse reactions to medications, hemophilia, leukemia, liver disease, and nutritional deficiencies. All berries are rich in vitamin P or the bioflavonoids rutin and hesperidin. These nutrients are able to do on-site repair work of these damaged, miniscule blood vessels. When this happens, skin discoloration eventually ceases.

Multiple Sclerosis.   Some berries—currants, for example—contain small amounts of a triple unsaturated fatty acid known as gamma linoleic acid (GLA). This nutrient isn't found inside the body but must be supplied through the diet. It is essential to the production of a fatty protein substance called myelin, which encases the nerve fibers running from the brain through the spinal cord. Think of any electrical cord and you have a good idea of what I mean: a plastic coating (myelin) surrounds a copper wire inside (the nerve) which conducts power through it. When there is a deficiency of GLA in the diet, the body begins to turn on itself and an autoimmune situation develops in the form of multiple sclerosis which attacks this myelin, causing scarring (sclerosis).

Urinary Tract Infection.   There are infections that occur in the urinary tracts of children as well as adults. They usually affect the bladder and urethra (the tube through which urine flows from the body). Sometimes, however, the infection arises in or spreads to the kidneys. Berries, particularly cranberries, are especially useful therapy for this problem. As reported in *The Journal of Urology* (131:1013-1016, 1984), cranberry juice contains a couple of constituents that appear to make disease-carrying bacteria less likely to cling to the surface of bladder and urinary tract cells. It is the quinic and benzoic acids in the cranberries that produce hippuric acid in the body, which is a potent inhibitor of such bacterial adherence.

METHOD OF PREPARATION

Berries may be juiced when they are ripe and freshly picked. As mentioned in the very beginning of this section, one of the simplest solutions is to pour boiling hot water over the crushed berries and let them sit for a couple of hours before straining off the juice. For plumper, juicier berries, rubbing them over a colander or thick wire sieve will bring the juice out quickly enough.

If you're intending to juice them by machine, you can do so in a food blender or Vita-Mix. It's best though to add one cup of water for every cup of berries you intend to juice this way. The speed you select for doing this will depend in large part on the size and ripeness of the berry itself. Figure about 1 to 1-$\frac{1}{2}$ minutes for this procedure.

I've found that apple cider is a good medium to use in place of water sometimes for diluting berry juice. It gives the juice more nip and flavor. In the event that some berry juices might need to be sweetened up a little, use pure maple syrup for this instead of sugar. One-half teaspoon of syrup for a pint of juice is adequate.

Some berry juices may be a little too tart for sensitive taste buds. Their sharpness can be greatly modified with certain spices. I recommend ground allspice, cardamom, cinnamon, and cloves for this purpose.

The juice combinations I prefer are as follows: blac berry and boysenberry; black and red currant; blueberry and huckleberry; boysenberry and raspberry; cranberry and raspberry; elderberry and boysenberry; gooseberry and black or red currant; huckleberry and blueberry; black raspberry and blackberry; red raspberry and elderberry; strawberry and cranberry; strawberry and elderberry.

A Proven Flu Fighter.   Other fruit juices also go great with individual berry juices. A winning combination to fight the common cold and "stomach flu" is cranberry juice (one quart), one can each of frozen lemonade and limeade, and one quart gingerale. Combine the juices together in your Vita-Mix or food blender. Then add a little honey or pure maple syrup for sweetener. After this, add the gingerale and some crushed ice cubes. Blend for almost two minutes before pouring and drinking. Sip slowly through a plastic straw. This is also an ideal mix for reducing fevers.

Another use for different berry juices found to be quite popular in Europe many decades ago, was in the form of a sweet aromatic liquor known as a cordial. Berry cordials were most often employed in gastrointestinal problems, such as upset stomach, diarrhea, constipation, dizziness and headaches (due to indigestion or liver or gall bladder troubles), and loss of appetite.

One such trustworthy cordial was made from the juice of pressed ripe blackberries. One-half teaspoon of cinnamon, cloves, and nutmeg with two tablespoons of sugar (substitute brown sugar here for the white kind) would be added to the juice. This would be brought to a short boil on the stove, then permitted to get cold, after which time a little brandy was added. The nice thing about cordials is that very little is taken internally, thereby stretching the amount of berry juice used.

BRUSSELS SPROUTS JUICE

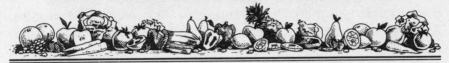

"Rejuvenating the Pancreas"

DESCRIPTION

Brussels sprouts (*Brassica oleracea, var. gemmifera*) are the newest members of the cabbage family, having been around in Europe for only about two hundred years. They grow on a very unusual yet attractive plant which, from a distance, looks a bit like a miniature green papaya tree. The leaves are up on the top of the plant and the tiny heads (called sprouts) completely surround the stalk. Brussels sprouts look like miniature heads of green cabbage.

Brussels sprouts thrive in cool, damp weather and for some reason are at their best when grown not too far from the ocean. Little wonder then that California is by far the number one source, but we import a fair amount from Mexico during the winter months. During the fall, until the first fairly heavy frost, Long Island, New York has a large, top quality crop, too.

Brussels sprouts are a biennial and come in two basic varieties: the Danish and the Long Island Improved. The smaller, firmer, and greener the sprout, the better the flavor. Soft, flabby ones, even if green, are less desirable than the hard, compact sprouts; and those with yellow leaves are undesirable.

NUTRITIONAL DATA

Four sprouts contain the following essential nutrients: 27 mg. calcium, 60 mg. phosphorus, 0.9 mg. iron, 8 mg. sodium, 229 mg. potassium, 440 I.U. vitamin A, trace amounts of B-complex vitamin, and 73 mg. of vitamin C.

As strange as it may seem, brussels sprouts which are harvested *after* the first real ground frost hits, are significantly higher in manganese and chromium, than those picked before the temperature drops. These two minerals are important for carbohydrate metabolism and maintaining normal blood sugar levels within the body.

THERAPEUTIC BENEFITS

Enrico C., an Italian by birth, came to America with his parents in the early 1950s when he was a boy. They settled down in the borough of Queens N.Y. His family brought with them their ethnic "love affair with food." "My mother used to cook all kinds of things, most of which were heavy in starch, often very oily, and usually very sweet," he told me.

When Enrico turned ten years of age, certain symptoms began to manifest themselves in his body. "It seemed like my growth suddenly stopped despite a hearty appetite," he recounted. He continued to list other changes: malabsorption, foul bulky stools, and clubbing of the fingers. "But when my bronchitis with a persistent cough and recurrent pneumonia set in, then my mama and papa became very worried," he said.

He was sent to a local hospital by their family physician for extensive tests. "I remember them poking different objects into me," he chuckled, "and giving me some stuff to drink [liquid barium] before they x-rayed the heck out of me. The prognosis for what I had—cystic fibrosis—looked pretty grim." The doctors told his parents that this disease was blocking Enrico's pancreatic ducts and that he needed replacement pancreatic juice and enzymes if he was to be given a 50-50 chance of surviving.

"Mama wasn't too crazy about what they had to offer," he mentioned, "so she consulted an old naturopathic doctor in the neighborhood for some medical assistance. He recommended to her that she get some small, firm brussels sprouts, picked after the first cold spell, and then run them through a hand-turned vegetable grinder and give me the juice to drink. She found this method pretty tiresome, so she switched to cooking them in water for an hour and then giving me the strained liquid to drink after it cooled.

"I got one cup of this in the afternoon and another at night before going to bed. She kept this up for about six months. Pretty soon most of my symptoms went away. I started growing again, putting on weight, had normal toilet activity, stopped my coughing, and got much better in my lungs. The only thing that took a little longer to straighten out were my fingers."

To this day, Enrico has had no recurring evidence of cystic fibrosis. He still includes brussels sprouts in his diet several times a week, though, "just to be on the safe side," he added.

Appetite Loss.   Just about everyone has experienced a short bout with anorexia at some time in his or her life. Stress, anxiety, fear, excitement, and emotional conflicts are among the many factors that can depress an individual's appetite. Almost any illness, ranging from the common cold to cancer and other potentially fatal disease, can cause temporary cessation of eating. So can smoking, alcohol, and many medications. Brussels sprouts contain valuable mineral salts such as potassium and sulphur, which promote the flow of greater saliva into the gut via the taste buds located along either side of the tounge and the olfactory senses within the nostrils. These sensory receptors send signals to the limbic portion or "pleasure center" of the brain, which, in turn, inspires the sensation for hunger.

Stunted Growth.   The physical condition of being abnormally un-dersized can be due to one of several different factors. A lack of sufficient growth hormones due to glandular dysfunction is one of these. A severe narrowing of the large artery arising from the base of the left ventricle of the heart, which prevents normal blood flow and nourishment to the rest of the growing body, is another reason. An inadequate development of the sexual organs, which produce certain hormones, is a third. And plain malnourishment, which deprives the body of essential vitamins, minerals, amino acids, and enzymes necessary for growth, is a fourth. I have noticed as an anthropologist that in those cultures which have access to plenty of sulphur-rich foods, their young children don't suffer very much from stunted growth. Since bussels sprouts contain sulphur, it will be of obvious value here. As to how the sulphur works in this regard, still remains a mystery.

METHOD OF PREPARATION

Wash and prepare the following combination of vegetables to be juiced together into a single drink: one-fourth piece red cabbage, one medium, peeled and topped carrot, six fresh brussels sprouts, eight string beans, one-half peeled cucumber, one-half Jerusalem artichoke, one-fourth Boston lettuce, and one bunch parsley. Drink this in one-half cup amounts every four hours *before* a meal.

CABBAGE JUICE

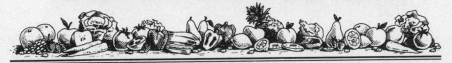

"Healing the Gastrointestinal Tract"

DESCRIPTION

The common heading cabbage (*Brassica oleracea, var. capitata Linn.*) produces a round, pointed, or flat head the first year and a seedstalk the second year. It is probably the most popular member of the cabbage family, being grown in all parts of the world. The wild form of cabbage probably was known to ancient people a long time before Christ, although it is uncertain whether the cabbage mentioned in ancient times was the heading type or the wild form having only a head of loose leaves. Its greatest development probably took place in Europe. The stem is short and terminates in a large bud, which is the edible portion of the plant. This bud or head can weigh anywhere from two to fifty pounds, depending on the type and variety.

Cabbage is a popular vegetable because it can be used as well in the raw state as in the preserved or cooked state. Its outer leaves are generally green, while the inner leaves are white. Vitamin nutrition is more abundant in the green leaves. It has a mild flavor, probably enjoyed by more people than that of any other vegetable. It is also an ideal food for animals, and people who have a flock of chickens find it an ideal green food for winter feeding.

Cabbage is divided into early or late, smooth- or crinkly-leaved, green or purple, and conical-, round-, or flat-headed varieties, as well as in different combinations.

NUTRITIONAL DATA

One cup of raw, shredded cabbage intended for cole slaw, yields the following nutrients: 116 mg. calcium, 31 mg. phosphorus, 0.6 mg. iron, 18 mg. sodium, 214 mg. potassium, 2,170 I.U. vitamin A, trace amounts of vitamin B-complex, and 18 mg. vitamin C.

In addition to this, cabbage contains a high amount of another very important mineral which we don't hear too much about — namely, sulphur. In fact, when cabbage is cooked, the odor you smell is the sulphur evaporating into the air.

Considerable research has been done with the sulphur compounds in cabbage and related members of the large *Brassica* family. Dr. Lee W. Wattenberg of the Department of Laboratory Medicine and Pathology at the University of Minnesota in Minneapolis, pioneered much of the work with a number of cruciferous plants. His studies, such as one published in the May, 1978 issue of *Cancer Research* (38:1410-13), have shown that brussels sprouts, cabbage, cauliflower and broccoli inhibit the development of harmful chemical carcinogens within the body. It's little wonder then that physician Donald R. Germann, M.D. recommended the following sulphur-rich vegetables in his book, *The Anti-Cancer Diet* (New York: Wideview Books, 1980): brussels sprouts, cabbage, broccoli, cauliflower, spinach, turnips, lettuce, celery, and dill.

In 1947, the *Journal of Nutrition* (23:602–12) presented compelling evidence to show that the sulphur compounds in cabbage, garlic, and onion almost neutralize the toxic effects of excess cobalt, nickel, and copper in the human body.

Even earlier than this, in the October, 1923 issue of *Proceedings of the Society for Experimental Biology and Medicine* (21:16–18), it was reported that cabbage, celery, and lettuce "contain both blood-sugar increasing and blood-sugar decreasing substances," which were attributed mostly to sulphur compounds.

More recent research has determined that the sulphur amino acids in cabbage are very good for lowering elevated serum cholesterol, calming agitated nerves and anxiety, lifting a depressed spirit and helping to bring on a good night's rest.

Maurice Mességué, France's most famous folk healer, mentioned the benefits of cabbage sulphur in his book *Mon Herbier de Santé* (Paris: Laffont/Tchou, 1975) by recalling this little incident:

> "A middle-aged woman suffering from chronic bronchitis once came to consult me, and I prescribed for her large quantities of cabbage, either in soup, salads, or in juice. In two months she was cured."

Another curious thing about sulphur is that it stimulates the production of friendly microflora within the colon. When cabbage fiber was ingested by six volunteers and later excreted, their stools showed that it had been extensively broken down and that there was a lot more microbial growth than in stools of subjects consuming wheat bran, which didn't digest as easily. (This report appeared in *Nature* 284:283–284, March 20, 1980.)

Thus, we can see from the array of evidence presented here that sulphur is an extremely vital nutrient to the overall health and well-being of our bodies.

THERAPEUTIC BENEFITS

I remember the late Seventh-Day Adventist physician, M. Charlotte Holmes, M.D., telling me back in 1988 that "raw or cooked cabbage juice and fermented sauerkraut and its juice are some of the best therapeutic agents for healing complaints of the gastrointestinal tract." She especially liked sauerkraut juice because "it contains lactic acid that is very soothing to the intestines." "I recommend it all the time to my female patients who are expecting; it helps them get over their morning sickness very quickly."

She told of one desperate situation in Macon County, Georgia, which she successfully treated a number of years ago. "This man about 55 years of age was in dire straits with a duodenal ulcer," she began. "Before he came to see me, he was taking a bottle of antacid a day and pills to chew on in his truck. But even with these things, he still was in great agony. So much ulcer scar had built up inside of him that an operation was all but out of the question.

"He said to me, 'Doctor Holmes, you're my last resort!' I gave him raw, unfiltered, smelly cabbage juice to drink in ten ounce portions morning and night. Within three weeks his antacid consumption had dropped by 50 percent. About four months later his ulcer had completely healed. This is an old standby I'm never without; I'll take it over Tums® and Rolaids® any day," she concluded.

Fresh cabbage juice is very good for treating alcoholics suffering from liver and stomach problems. The *Journal of The American Medical Association* (178:869, Nov. 25, 1961) attributes the success of cabbage juice to the presence of small amounts of glutamine, an essential amino acid. *The Medical Journal of Australia* (December 15, 1979 and February 9, 1980) also verifies the success of cabbage juice in treating hangovers and peptic and duodenal ulcers due to excessive alcohol consumption. The articles in this journal point to the "vitamin U" and sulphur amino acids as being responsible for results elicited.

A very good summary of the many positive health benefits of cabbage may be found in the article, "Physiological effects of cabbage with reference to its potential as a dietary cancer-inhibitor and its use in ancient medicine," by Michael Albert-Puleo, which appeared in the *Journal of Ethnopharmacology* (9:261–272, 1983).

Cancer. An important study published in the *Journal of the National Cancer Institute* (61:709-14, September 1978) showed that men and women who consumed cabbage, Brussels sprouts, and broccoli on a fairly regular basis, had significantly decreased incidents of colo-rectal cancers. The sulphur compounds present in cabbage prevent food-ingested chemical carcinogens from combining to form mutated cells, which lead to tumors.

Cholesterol (Elevated). The *Journal of Nutritional Science and Vitaminology* (31:121-125, Jan–Feb 1985), a Japanese scientific publication, reported that the cholesterol levels fell in rats because of the sulphur-containing amino acids present in the food they ate. Since cabbage is rich in sulphur—you can even smell it when it's cooking—it can lower elevated plasma cholesterol.

Diabetes. A scientist named J. J. Lewis conducted some interesting experiments with rabbits in 1950. His two reports appeared in the

British Journal of Pharmacology (5:21-24; 455-460). He noted that: ". . . the blood sugar after one hour is significantly lower when cabbage extract is administered with solution of dextrose than when solution of dextrose is administered alone," and suggested that "the extract appears to slow down and prolong dextrose absorption." This is mainly due to the water-holding fiber in cabbage pulp, while the sulphur in the juice extract manifests "an insulin-like activity," he noted.

METHOD OF PREPARATION

Some juice advocates and a few juice books suggest mixing raw cabbage juice with either pineapple or pear juice to improve the taste and create unusual flavors. However, I'm reminded of something which the late Finnish nutritionist, Paavo Airola, Ph.D., N.D. told me about fifteen years ago at a National Health Federation convention in Phoenix, Arizona. He said, "Only under unusual circumstances should you ever combine vegetable and fruit juices together. They're incompatible with each other and can only create more trouble than good!"

My recommendation is that raw cabbage juice be combined with equal amounts of celery, endive, watercress, or parsley juice. Half of a medium-sized cabbage should yield about a cup of juice. For an interesting color and taste variation, juice one-quarter each of white and red cabbage. Any juicer with a shredder/blade or rotating cutter on a shaft is good for obtaining cabbage juice.

Keep in mind that frequent consumption of cabbage can deplete iodine levels in the body, thereby weakening the thyroid gland. Be sure to take ample kelp (a seaweed), (2) tablets or capsules, or season your food with it (available in powdered or granulated forms from any health food store).

CANTALOUPE JUICE

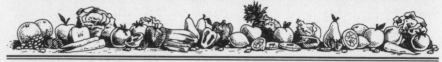

"Cooling Beverage for Fevers"

DESCRIPTION

Cantaloupe or muskmelon (*Cucumis melo cantalupensis*) grows on a bushy plant with long outreaching vines. Cantaloupe comes with a hard ridged or warty rind and reddish orange flesh inside. There are several varieties to choose from:

• The ambrosia is the standard-size fruit and makes one of the best eating cantaloupes around;

• The bushwhopper is another cantaloupe, which grows on a compact plant only 2-½ feet wide;

• The Minnesota midget is a small, sweet cantaloupe that ripens in only two months and has 3-foot vines;

• The oval chaca hybrid grows on large vines and is quite resistant to fusarium wilt and powdery mildew that can seriously affect other kinds of cantaloupe;

• The short and sweet cantaloupe grows on a small, bushy plant that is resistant to heat, drought, and powdery mildew.

To produce sweet-tasting cantaloupe, the melon plant needs a long, hot growing season. If you plant them in a cool summer climate, you can increase the heat around the plant by letting the vines run on concrete or by simply spreading black plastic under the vines in the vegetable garden. If you let the vines cascade over a rocky embankment, the rocks will hold the heat at night and achieve the same effect.

NUTRITIONAL DATA

One-half cantaloupe contains the following nutrients: 38 mg. calcium, 44 mg. phosphorus, 1.1 mg. iron, 33 mg. sodium, 682 mg. potassium, 9,240 I.U. vitamin A, 1.6 mg. niacin, and 90 mg. vitamin C.

A different analysis of the nutritional content of cantaloupe and honeydew melons appeared in the *Journal of Food Science* (50:136–138, 1985). It showed an average of the following additional nutrients in milligram measurements per 100 grams of cantaloupe: 12.69 magnesium, 0.03 manganese, 0.05 copper, 0.10 zinc, 0.003 cobalt, and 0.005 chromium.

The study also showed that cantaloupes purchased at periods near maximum availability had "significantly higher…levels of niacin, riboflavin, thiamine, ascorbic acid, folacin, and chromium compared to those purchased near minimum availability." This suggests that cantaloupe *in season* is better for you nutritionally, than melon out of season.

THERAPEUTIC BENEFITS

Barbara Wilson, R.N., who has worked with the Peace Corps in various locations in the South Pacific and is a frequent contributor to *Folk Medicine Journal*, related this episode to me awhile back.

> "While making various house calls for a clinic I work out of sometimes in South Los Angeles, I came upon one impoverished Vietnamese family whose seven-year-old daughter was extremely sick. They spoke very broken English and I spoke no Vietnamese, yet somehow we managed to communicate pretty well under the circumstances.
>
> "The parents gave me to understand that their little girl had been bitten by a rodent of some kind. In examining the child, she showed all of the classical signs of rat-bite fever: a relapsing fever, chills, headache, severe joint pain, swollen lymph nodes, and a maculopapular rash on her extremities.
>
> "Because the child was too sick and frail, I didn't want to run the risk of giving her any antibiotics which could have had an unfavorable

reaction in her very weakened condition. I went to a nearby super-market and bought some ripe cantaloupes. I had the woman working in the deli area peel the melons after I paid for them at the checkout counter. I then persuaded her to run them through her juicer, which she used in the morning to make freshly squeezed orange juice and which had already been cleaned out. After giving her the reason for this, she gladly honored my request, feeling a satisfaction, I suppose, in being able to help a sick child.

"I took close to a quart of this cantaloupe juice back to the Vietnamese residence and gave the young girl half a cupful, which she slowly sipped. I instructed her parents to give their daughter one half cupful of this juice every few hours. I did this with a lot of arm and hand gestures and very simply pronounced words they could understand.

"I returned to their tiny apartment several days later, and discovered their daughter running around outside with her friends. She was full of life and energy again and no one would have ever guessed just how sick she had been a few days prior to this. Her recovery speaks volumes in support of the remarkable refrigerant properties of canta-loupe for any type of major or minor fever."

Crohn's disease.   Regional enteritis (another name for this autoim-mune disorder) is a chronic condition characterized by inflammation of the lower segment of the small intestine (known as the ileum) or the large intestine (colon), or both. It can occur at any age, but is most common in young men and women. When inflamed areas heal, they may become fibrous, leading to a narrowing of the bowel. This, in turn, can produce partial or total obstruction of the intestinal flow. Cantaloupe is incredibly rich in beta-carotene. This provitamin A, along with trace elements like magnesium, manganese, zinc, and chromium present in the melon juice, can effectively reduce this inflammation and restore natural health to injured mucosal tissue. The natural sugars and enzymes present in cantaloupe exert a laxative effect in the colon.

Upset Stomach.   Distress in the digestive tract can be due to excess worrying, eating in a hurry without proper chewing, spicy foods, alcohol, drugs, ulcer, or an accumulation of intestinal gas. Some cantaloupe juice works well for this complaint because its natural sugars and enzymes have a settling effect on the gut.

METHOD OF PREPARATION

Select a ripe cantaloupe. Cut it in half, scoop out the seeds, and wash the inside out under the sink tap. Then peel and cut into several smaller sections lengthwise. Then quarter these width-wise into small chunks or enough to yield about two cups (which will make approximately two-third cup of juice). Juice the cantaloupe and set aside.

Wash out the container and place back on the machine. Combine four teaspoons cashew nut butter, one tablespoon each of finely chopped black mission figs and pitted dates, two-third cup soymilk, one-fourth teaspoon dark honey or blackstrap molasses, one-half teaspoon pure almond extract, and one-half cup coarsely crushed ice cubes.

Blend on high speed for about one and one-half minutes. Then add the cantaloupe juice and continue blending for another one and one-half minutes until smooth like velvet to the tongue. Not only will this make a very therapeutic drink for reducing even the highest fever, but it is also tasty enough to give to even the most discriminating youngster or fussy adult. It is truly "mighty good tasting medicine in a glass!"

CARROT JUICE

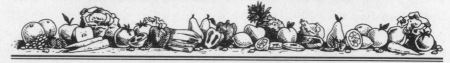

"Prescription for Improved Vision"

DESCRIPTION

Carrots (*Daucus carota, var. sativa*) are among the most popular and nutritious vegetables grown. The smaller and earlier types, which are of high quality, are grown for human consumption, while the large-rooted late varieties are grown for stock feed. The carrot, as we know it, is supposed to have originated from the wild carrot, often called Queen Anne's lace. This happens to be one of the worst weeds we have to contend with, especially in abandoned meadow land. In cultivated ground it is not as much trouble.

The varieties of carrots may be grouped into six distinct types according to shape and size of the corresponding root:

1. The French forcing or earliest short horn is the smallest and earliest carrot that is grown. The root is almost as thick as it is long, has a golden, orange-red color, and makes a nice, colorful juice.

2. The oxheart type, of orange-red color, is one third longer than it is broad and tapers gradually towards the tip. The small to medium-sized roots, approximating three inches in length, are good for bunch carrots but are better suited for cut carrots for storing.

3. The Chantenay type is probably the most important for the canning industry and as a bushel carrot for storage. It has a better juice quality than the oxheart type has.

4. The Danvers half-long is just what its name implies. It is not so thick as the Chantenay and grows to about seven inches in length, or about two-thirds the length of the true Danvers type which has given way to other long slender varieties. This half-long type has been very popular in the New England states, where it was grown along with bushel carrots. It tapers gradually to a rather sharp point in contrast to the Chantenay type.

5. The Nantes is a half-long type and probably should be included in the Danvers group, but because of its characteristic shape and particularly high quality, it deserves special consideration. It is an ideal bunching carrot and is generally grown in the midwestern states in the market-gardening sections. It grows to a length of eight inches and is cylindrical in shape, being almost as broad near the tip as it is at the butt end. It is much higher in sugar content than some of the other varieties previously mentioned. Its color is an orange-red. This makes the best carrot juice in terms of flavor, quick energy and a wakeup "bugle-call-in-the-ear" which snaps the liver to immediate attention. For mineral content, though, the Chantenay type seems to be higher in things like calcium and potassium than is the Nantes.

6. The long, slender type is represented by such varieties as Hutchinson, Morses Bunching, Imperator, and Streamliner. These carrots average eleven inches in length and are of particularly high quality. When fully mature, the roots are orange-red in color. Most of the carrots grown for market on the West Coast are varieties of this group. This type needs a deep soil that is well limed in order to produce enough sugar and minerals to make its juicing worthwhile. I've tasted carrot juice in some Southern California health food stores made from this type and other juice in several midwestern health food stores made from the Nantes type, and I can verify that there is a world of taste and nutritional difference in both kinds. Ideally, one should be able to juice the Chantenay and Nantes types together. Now there's a winning juice combination for sure!

NUTRITIONAL DATA

One carrot $7\text{-}\frac{1}{2}$ inches long and $1\text{-}\frac{1}{8}$ inches in diameter, yields the following nutrients: 27 mg. calcium, 26 mg. phosphorus, 0.5 mg. iron, 34 mg. sodium, 246 mg. potassium, 7,930 I.U. vitamin A, trace amounts of vitamin B-complex, and 6 mg. vitamin C.

Carrots

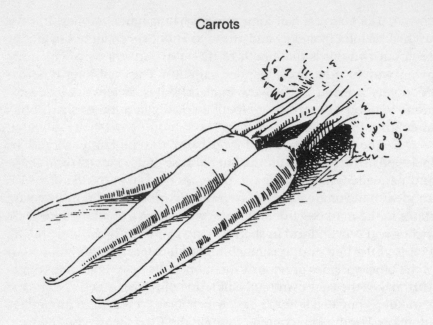

Another nutritional analysis done by Lancaster Laboratories for the Vita-Mix Corporation, listed these additional nutrients per 100 grams of carrot juice: 8.2 mg. magnesium and 0.2 ppm (parts per million) chromium. The sugar profile broke down as follows: fructose 1.5 percent by weight, dextrose 0.8 percent by weight, sucrose 1.9 percent by weight, maltose 0.3 percent by weight, and lactose 0.5 percent by weight. Total sugar content was 4 percent by weight.

In neither analysis were the specific types of carrot used ever identified.

THERAPEUTIC BENEFITS

Every so often I get to Phoenix, Arizona, where I generally do a Saturday morning live talk show with my friend and colleague, Dr. Bob Martin on radio station KFYI-AM. Afterwards, a mutual friend of ours, Irvin "Herb" Markovitz has me over to his Cinema Park Super Health Foods store for a couple of hours to do book autographs and answer customers' health questions.

The last time such an event took place, over 200 people lined up outside to buy my books and get a chance to visit with me. Among them was a young woman named Cherylnn, age 37, who worked in a local architect's office. She suffered from eye strain, "floaters" in the eyes and occasional moments of blurred vision.

My advice to her was this: "Bathe the eyes once a day with a weak solution of boric acid powder (one-half teaspoon) and warm chamomile tea (one cup). Drink a full glass of mixed greens (one-fourth part) and carrot juice (three-fourth part) every other day after doing this." I gave her my card and asked if she would please contact me in the event she needed further assistance with her problem.

About two months later, a note arrived in the mail, reminding me of the incident and identifying the writer as the woman I had helped. She stated that within a week her eyes were much better from following the simple recommendations I had made. And within three weeks' time, she was even able to drive in the dark again (something which had been a problem for her to do before this treatment began).

This is a real testimony to the power of carrot juice for treatment of vision.

Complexion Problems.   Many young people in their teens and early twenties are often bothered with things like pimples, whiteheads, and blackheads. Older adults may be plagued with more serious skin disorders such as boils, cysts, and abscesses. If none of these eruptions appear, then the skin may be rough and dry, and have a leathery feel to it. All of these complexion problems are mainly due to poor diet and bad lifestyle habits (smoking, alcoholism, drug addiction). These things result in an extreme acid condition of the blood. Carrot juice is rich enough in potassium to help neutralize this excess acid and contains an incredible amount of vitamin A to assist the liver in removing such toxins from the body.

Heavy Metal Accumulations.   Most of us are exposed to heavy metals in the air we breathe, the water we drink, and the pesticide-sprayed leafy greens we eat. Other exposure may come from certain cookware we prepare our foods in, or the consumption of peeled paint flakes from walls by small and curious children in old tenement dwellings. It is interesting to note that in the former Soviet Union, factory workers in occupational environments that exposed them to many toxic metals, were routinely prescribed foods which have the ability to remove such things from the body very quickly. According to *The American Journal of Clinical Nutrition* (42:746-48, October 1985), carrot juice, green peas, potatoes, cabbage, tomato puree, cranberries, and other unspecified "fresh fruits" can pull these heavy metals from fatty tissue where they reside, bind them up, and discharge them from the system.

Lupus Erythematosus. Systemic lupus erythematosus (SLE) is an inflammatory disease that can damage connective tissue throughout the body, including tissue in the joints, muscles, skin, kidneys, heart, lungs, and nervous system. It is an unusual form of arthritis that afflicts mostly women. In fact, women outnumber men with this autoimmune disorder by a ratio of more than 9 to 1. For unknown reasons, lupus is also more common in African-Americans and in some Asian and Native American groups than in Caucasians or Hispanics. While SLE usually lasts a lifetime, it can be remedied with high amounts of vitamin A, mineral salts, and natural carbohydrates. Carrot juice meets all of this criteria very nicely. But so as not to subject the liver to an excessive amount of carrot juice, which would tend to turn the skin a yellowish-orange hue, it's recommended that the juice be diluted with an equal amount of liquid chlorophyll of some kind.

METHOD OF PREPARATION

One of the most delicious drinks I've ever made for improving failing eyesight calls for several ingredients ordinarily never blended together. However, I'm always one for experimentation and the discovery of new things, which is precisely how I came up with this concoction in the first place.

Wash and scrub (but don't peel) one medium Chantenay and one small to medium Nantes carrots (see *Description* section for details on both types). Next, wash and scrub (but don't peel) one small red beet. Remove the leaves and use them in a salad or lightly steam for cooked greens or juice when you need liquid chlorophyll.

Cut the carrots into smaller pieces and juice them first. Set the carrot juice aside. Then cut the beet into several sections and juice it. Combine both juices, along with one-half cup unwhipped cream and one-half teaspoon each of pure vanilla flavor and pure maple syrup. Blend in together for two minutes on variable low speed.

The exotic flavor and deep rich color which such a juice presents to the eye and palate are indescribable but certainly worth every single sip. The only dilemma may be in resisting the urge to have a second or even third glass of this juice mixture.

CELERY JUICE

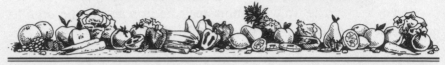

"Relief for Eczema and Psoriasis"

DESCRIPTION

Celery (*Apium graveolens*) is grown for its edible leaf-stalks, which are fleshy and tender and have a nut-like flavor when blanched. Although the green, unblanched celery has a slightly bitter flavor, it is becoming more popular every year as a favorite snack item in restaurant salad bars and in party hors d'oeuvres. Much of the selection of the cultivated varieties was made possibly during the 15th century from a wild, bitter, southern European plant once used as a medicine and as an herb for flavoring purposes. In its wild state, celery is a marsh plant with hollow stalks, but the cultivated varieties have been developed for the firmness of the leafstalks.

Celery varieties are grouped into two types, the yellow and the green. The yellow or self-blanching type is represented by a golden or white plume and by easy blanching. The green type is represented by Golden Crisp and Giant Pascal.

NUTRITIONAL DATA

One stalk of celery has the following nutrients in it: 16 mg. calcium, 11 mg. phosphorus, 0.1 mg. iron, 50 mg. sodium, 136 mg. potassium, 110 I.U. vitamin A, trace amounts of some B-complex vitamins, and

Celery

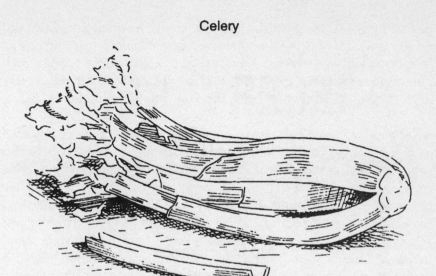

4 mg. vitamin C. Another nutritional analysis shows that celery has appreciable amounts of magnesium in a range of 27–32 mg. per celery stalk.

THERAPEUTIC BENEFITS

King Henry VIII (1491–1547) was one of England's more illustrious— if not somewhat infamous—monarchs. His social relations, especially with women, left much to be desired. In fact, some of his many ex-wives were either imprisoned, banished, or beheaded, depending on his mood at the time their separate fates were being decided.

Henry also suffered from a bad complexion, which may have been one of the reasons some of his wives shunned him whenever they could. Because of his gluttonous habits and preponderance for meats, pastries, wines, and ales, his forehead, face, arms, hands, and legs would often break out in varying degrees of rash.

Various ointments and other topical medications proved of little avail. One of the court physicians heard about a local herbalist curing similar skin problems with the juice of *smallage* (what was then called celery). He obtained sufficient quantities of this herb and had the kitchen cooks extract juice from the leaves and stems by amply pounding them. He gave this juice to Henry in small amounts, and within days the king's complexion improved, only to return to its former condition whenever he returned to eating those foods which contributed to it. But the good doctor kept pouring enough celery juice down him so that, at least, the rash was held in check.

Allergies. It has been my own experience, both personal as well as through observation, that there is a strong connection between sugar intake and allergic reactions. Whenever I begin consuming one or two majool dates a day, my allergy to the cat I keep in my office becomes more profound. Immediate and prolonged sneezing and the itching of my eyes becomes very apparent. When I make myself some fresh celery juice and drink $\frac{1}{2}$ cup for several days straight, these symptoms soon abate. I find it's the strong mineral salts in celery, which makes my blood very alkaline. When this happens my allergies go into remission almost as quickly as they started up when I commenced eating a few very tasty dates.

Blood Poisoning. This is a condition in which bacteria infects the blood. In mild cases, there may be no symptoms; in general, though, it can be quite serious. Stepping on a rusty nail, allowing dirt to get into a wound, an extensive burn, urinary tract infection, and hospitalization for surgery are some of the underlying causes for sepsis or septicemia (blood poisoning). The high amount of mineral salts in celery make it very alkaline. The bacteria responsible for blood poisoning thrives better in acidic conditions than they do in an alkaline environment. The presence of celery in the body helps to dilute their potential harm.

Hyperactivity and Attention Deficit Disorder. Frequent   restlessness and an inability to focus on something for very long, constitute hyperactivity. The more preferred term these days, however, is attention deficit disorder (ADD) to describe such overly active kids. Factors believed to be involved in ADD are: overproduction of adrenal hormones; impaired mental function; overactive thyroid; stress; artificial colors and flavors in food, beverages, and candy; adverse drug reactions; and high sugar intake. The late Benjamin Goldfein, M.D., a California pediatrician, believed that most of these things caused an excess acid condition in the blood of the hyperactive child. By removing them and giving the child mineral-rich foods instead, great improvements could soon be noticed in behavior patterns. Celery has been one of those foods recommended by some nutritionists and doctors specializing in treating children with ADD.

METHOD OF PREPARATION

Because straight celery juice may be a little sharp to the taste buds and slightly overpowering to the liver, it may be a good idea to mix it with a little carrot juice. One of the best combinations for curing eczema and psoriasis is to use a mixture of celery, Swiss chard, and cucumber juices diluted with a little carrot juice.

Wash (but don't peel) four medium-sized carrots (which yield about a cup of juice). Separate and clean two stalks of celery (equivalent to one-half cup of juice) under tap water. Wash a small unpeeled cucumber (one-half cup juice) with soap and water, then rinse. Next, wash a small bunch of Swiss chard (one and one-half tablespoons).

Separately juice each of these items and set aside in different cups. Then combine everything together in your food blender for one minute. The mixture yields a little over two cups. Drink separately from meals.

CHERRY JUICE

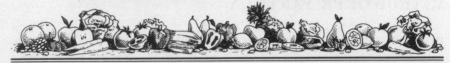

"Quick and Easy Relief for Arthritis and Gout"

DESCRIPTION

Cherries (*Prunus avium*) are drupes that are very closely related to plums and more distantly related to peaches and nectarines. They are tasty, colorful, nutritious, and require no preparation. If cherries have a single flaw, it is that they are available for an all too short period of time. The cherry season is short and sweet.

Although cherries originated in the Middle East and have been cultivated for thousands of years in both European and Eastern countries, by far the biggest producer, user, and exporter of cherries is the United States.

In the purchase of almost any other fresh fruit, there are several good varieties to choose from, but when it comes to cherries, it's a one-horse race. The Bing variety is in a class all by itself. The rest of the cherry varieties are either also-rans or never-rans. The Bing is the tastiest, firmest, meatiest, and largest cherry grown.

There are two light-colored or white varieties of cherries—the Napoleons (Royal Anne's) and the Raniers. These attractive cherries are cream-colored and sport a red cheek. They have good size and a fairly good flavor. The white cherries are not as firm as the dark cherries, are more fragile, are bruised easily and have a short shelf life. They have never become very popular possibly because just as some people will buy only red-skinned apples, many people expect cherries to be red.

NUTRITIONAL DATA

Cherries are a great snack when you're on a diet, since they contain a mere 82 calories per cup serving (unpitted, of course). Furthermore, the same cup contains: 32 mg. calcium, 28 mg. phosphorus, 0.6 mg. iron, 3 mg. sodium, 277 mg. potassium, 160 I.U. vitamin A, some B-complex vitamins, and 15 mg. vitamin C.

THERAPEUTIC BENEFITS

At a Whole Life Expo in Pasadena, California in March of 1993, I met a retired insurance executive named Sam Johnson. He was one of many who packed the small lecture hall intended for 100 but somehow managing to accommodate almost double that number.

In my discussion of "Food Cures for the Nineties," I mentioned an episode from my childhood with an old junk peddler named Ray Ivie. My father and I used to go to many of the same rummage sales that he went to. I still can picture the old gent in my memory dragging that old gunny sack of his around and popping into it whatever items he thought were a bargain and pleased his fancy.

I told my attentive audience that he often complained of severe gout which he suffered in his ankles and knees; so much, in fact, that sometimes he couldn't even shuffle without grimacing and hollering in great pain.

One time he asked my father, "Jake, do you know of anything I can take for this?" Whereupon, my father suggested that he try drinking cherry juice. Well, instead of juicing them while they were still raw, he had his wife cook a pot of cherries for him. She then strained the liquid off and allowed it to cool. Mr. Ivie drank several cups of this each day. Within five days, he claimed, when he later saw us again at another garage sale, the pain and swelling had subsided enough that he could now "dance a jig and think nuthin' of it."

This account prompted Mr. Johnson to share a similar story with me afterwards. He had been bothered for years with lingering arthritis in his hands and wrists, making the usual burden of paperwork that his business generated, extremely difficult to complete.

One day he stopped by a highway fruit stand and, tempted by the appearance of some ripe cherries, decided to buy a pound to snack on as he drove to an insurance meeting some distance away.

"I really didn't notice the effects the fruit had on me," he recounted, "until I started using my pen. That's when it occurred to me that the usual pains just weren't there! I didn't give much thought to it after that, until the same pains returned a few days later. I thought back on those cherries and figured I'd better get some more of them."

This time he decided to make juice out of them instead of eating them whole. He found a rather novel way to get the pits out, he said. "I would put several into my mouth," he explained, "chew them just enough to spit the pits out, then put them into an empty cottage cheese container. After it was full, I ran them through our juicer and drank one and one-half glasses of the liquid I got. But I wouldn't recommend this method of getting the pits out for others around you, who might raise some loud objections to sharing your saliva," he laughed.

While his method of pit removal leaves something to be desired, it saved him a lot of manual labor having to cut each cherry with a paring knife and scraping the stone out that way. "As long as I drink three cups of cherry juice a week, my arthritis remains under control," he happily admitted. He freezes quite a few cherries when they're no longer in season, or else he buys some cherry juice concentrate from a local health food store and dilutes it according to label instructions. When worst comes to worst and neither of these is available, he's discovered that cherry-flavored cough syrup helps alleviate the pain to some small degree.

Acne Vulgaris.   Prolonged storage of toxins within the body, necessitate occasional breakouts through the skin in different places to relieve some of the buildup. Acne is one way in which the body reacts to so much internal poison. Cherry juice just happens to be a very effective blood cleanser for getting rid of accumulated waste materials. When a reduction takes place, skin problems soon begin to clear up of their own accord.

Rheumatism.   This is an obsolete term for a nonspecific disorder of the joints, slow in progress, producing a painful thickening and contraction of the fibrous structures. Rheumatism interferes with physical motion and causes deformity. Outdated medical texts of the late 19th century used to recommend cherry juice as an effective agent for reducing joint pain and inflammation. It accomplishes this by crystallized deposits of uric acid waste, which have accumulated in the joints over a lengthy period of time.

Skin Conditions.   Stress, poor diet, and substance abuse create a state of toxemia within the body. Cherries are a natural cleansing agent to help flush such acid poisons from the system by stimulating activity in the kidneys, bladder, and colon where most discharge of wastes takes place.

METHOD OF PREPARATION

Wash one pound of Bing cherries in a large colander under running water. Pick off the stems, rewash, and set aside.

Bring two quarts of water to a rapid boil, then reduce the heat to a lower setting. Place one handful of cherries in a large fine-mesh wire strainer with a long handle to it. Immerse them in the boiling water and retain there for *no more* than three minutes. Remove and drain the excess water away.

Next, place these cherries on top of a clean piece of linen, cloth diaper, or old bed sheet. Cover with another piece of similar size cloth after the cherries have been evenly spread out. Go over them lightly with a rolling pin, applying just enough pressure to squish out the pits, but not hard enough to remove the juice.

Uncover and remove by hand those remaining few which may still have pits in them. Set this batch aside and proceed as before until all of the cherries have been pitted in this manner.

They are now ready to be run through your juicer. One pound of ripe cherries yields nearly a full glass of juice.

CHERVIL JUICE

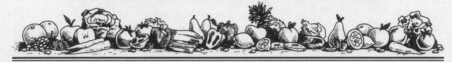

"Something Good for the Gall Bladder"

DESCRIPTION

There are two chervils, the annual and the biennial. The salad chervil (*Anthriscus cerefolium*) is the annual and is grown for its foliage, and in some sections of Europe was used as a pot herb. It is a native of the Caucasus, southern Russia, and western Asia. It has a parsley-type of foliage and the plant grows about 18 inches tall. The leaves are used for flavoring soups and meat dishes.

The parsnip-rooted chervil (*Chaerophyllium tuberosum*) is a biennial. It makes a rosette of leaves and fleshy taproot the first year and produces seed the second year. The roots are used very much like carrots. They resemble the carrot in shape and are brownish in color, while the flesh is yellow. The foliage is somewhat coarser than the salad chervil's. Both plants are highly esteemed by Europeans.

NUTRITIONAL DATA

Dried salad chervil contains the following nutrients for an edible portion weighing 100 grams: 1,346 mg. calcium, 31.95 mg. iron, 130 mg. magnesium, 450 mg. phosphorus, 4,740 mg. potassium, 83 mg. sodium, 8.80 mg. zinc, 1.225 mg. vitamin B_6, and undetermined amounts of vitamins A, B-complex, C, E, K, and P.

THERAPEUTIC BENEFITS

Mary Rigdon of Suffolk, England taught mathematics in a private boarding school for girls. She began experiencing an agonizing, colicky pain that started high in her abdomen and eventually began shooting up towards her right shoulder blade. Soon followed other symptoms such as sweating, occasional nausea, and vomiting, and an inability to keep still. She consulted with a local homeopathic physician, who diagnosed her problem as a severe attack of gall-stones.

The regimen prescribed for her consisted of the following plant medicinals: Extractum Taraxacum Liquor (an alcohol extract of dandelion root), one-half to one dram three times daily; boiled chicory root tea, one cup twice daily; and chervil leaf (*Anthriscus cerefolium*) juice, one-half cup twice daily in between meals.

She was also advised to lay off all greasy and sugary foods and instead to eat those things which were more beneficial to the system, such as whole grain cereals and breads, salads, fruits, and nuts. The doctor who used alternative medicine to treat her condition also suggested that she drink six large glasses of water every day.

Within a week's time, she reported feeling better and was able to resume her full teaching schedule without further discomfort. She, however, changed her eating habits and stayed with a diet that promoted good health. This information was relayed to me by a British colleague of mine familiar with the case.

Liver Problems.   The liver is one major organ of the body which is continually assaulted with a wide variety of chemicals present in the food we eat, the beverages we drink, and the drugs which many people routinely take. If any other organ were regularly subjected to such abuse for an extended period, it would, most likely, stop working.   Fortunately though, the liver is capable of regenerating itself. Chervil contains those components like chlorophyll, mineral salts, vitamins, and enzymes necessary for this regrowth transformation.

Spleen Pain and Inflammation.   The spleen is a large vascular lymphatic organ lying in the upper part of the abdominal cavity on the left side, between the stomach and diaphragm. It is composed of white and red pulp matter. It is a blood-forming organ in early life and a storage organ for red corpuscles. In the spleen may also be found a large number of immune defense scavenger cells called macrophages. They work like city street sweeping machines or the video game Pac-Man, gobbling up bacterial debris. For this reason the spleen acts as a blood filter. Sometimes, however, the spleen can become swollen and inflamed from overwork or infection. Chervil root and leaf have a definite affinity with this body organ in several different ways. Some of the nutrient contents help to fight whatever infection may be present, while certain chemical constituents soothe and relieve painful inflammation.

METHOD OF PREPARATION

While not as well known as other vegetables, chervil is still a very useful item for all gall bladder, kidney, and liver disorders. In Europe, it is used much more frequently than it is in the U.S. I recommend a combination of chervil, dark Romaine lettuce, and dandelion greens —equal parts of each—as a terrific tonic for problems in these three organs of the body. The leaves of each should be thoroughly washed before juicing them.

As an added health bonus, you should include the yellow flowering tops of dandelion. They are incredibly high in beta-caro-tene, ascorbic acid, bioflavonoids, and iron, all of which does the gall bladder and liver much good. In the event that the resulting juice is a little bitter on account of the dandelion tops, then add some carrot juice to the mixture to sweeten things up a bit, or else add some tomato or V-8® juice to give the drink more of an alkaline flavor. By stirring in a half teaspoon of powdered or granulated kelp (a seaweed) if you're using tomato or V-8® juice and squeezing in a little lemon or lime juice, you'll have a lip-smacking drink that will satisfy all of your cravings for salty snacks.

When juicing chervil, Romaine lettuce and dandelion greens, you need not do each one separately but can juice them all together. Then juice your carrot or tomato by itself, and combine with the other three afterwards.

CHICORY-ENDIVE JUICES

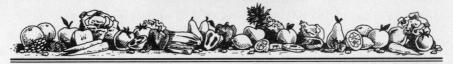

"A Great Combo for Osteoporosis"

DESCRIPTION

Chicory (*Cichorium intybus*) is often called endive or French endive and is grown for its tender though somewhat bitter salad leaves by forcing the roots. The roots themselves are, likewise, harvested then dried and ground into a powder as an adulterant for some brands of coffee. It most likely originated in Asia, but it is generally grown more in Europe than here in the United States.

It is a perennial plant that in its wild state grows along roadsides in the temperate regions of Europe and Asia. Chicory produces a nice rosette of leaves and a big fleshy root the first year. In the second year, it sends up a tall multi-branched seedstalk, covered with solitary, axillary, compound flowers of an attractive deep blue color.

Endive (*Cichorium endivia*) is a close relative of chicory and is either an annual or biennial salad plant. It forms a heavy rosette of curled and cut leaves. It is a native of the East Indies and has been grown for many years as a salad plant. The second year it produces a seedstalk somewhat similar to wild chicory. This type of endive is often sold in supermarket produce sections under the more familiar term of escarole. There are two types; the narrow-and the broad-leaf.

NUTRITIONAL DATA

One head of chicory yields the following essential nutrients: 10 mg. calcium, 11 mg. phosphorus, 0.3 mg. iron, 4 mg. sodium, 97 mg. potassium and undetermined but high amounts of vitamins C and magnesium with trace amounts of some B-complex vitamins.

One cup of escarole or endive, cut or broken into small pieces, contains these nutrients: 41 mg. calcium, 27 mg. phosphorus, 0.9 mg. iron, 7 mg. sodium, 147 mg. potassium, 1,650 I.U. vitamin A, 2.3 mg. niacin, 45 mg. vitamin C and close to 312 mg. magnesium.

THERAPEUTIC BENEFITS

Lillian Franck came over from the "Old Country" many decades ago and settled down in New York City, where she has resided the past 52 years in relatively good health. I met this spry and sharp little lady at the New Life Expo convention held in April of 1993. She took in my noontime lecture on "The Management of Pain with Foods and Herbs."

Afterwards, she came to the Light Energy exhibit where I was selling some of my books and answering people's personal health questions. When her turn came, she told me what she had done for her own osteoporosis.

From several local Korean markets in her neighborhood, she purchases fresh chicory and endive or escarole. Then in her apartment she washes them thoroughly before juicing in her Vita-Mix. Because of the strong flavor, she usually dilutes it with a little carrot or beet juice, either of which is sweet enough to take the slightly bitter edge away.

Mrs. Franck, who turned 86 in July, 1993, informed me that after drinking *one cup* of this combination each day for six months, her osteoporosis has all but disappeared. She thinks the calcium, potassium, phosphorus, and magnesium in both vegetables helped to significantly strengthen her bones. "I'd prescribe this to anybody," she laughed, "who is nearly as old as I am and would break like a china doll if they fell."

Fractures.   The strength of chicory and endive leaves is in their high magnesium contents. Consider magnesium to be "the glue" that holds calcium and phosphorus to the bones of the body. When there is insufficient magnesium, then there will inevitably be a loss of valuable calcium from the skeletal structure. Bone fractures mend well when an assortment of minerals and enzymes are present. But magnesium is the key critical to recovery. It is the stuff which keeps other nutrients "stuck" in place during the healing process.

Herniated Disc.   A structurally weak disk may become deformed (much like an old mattress). The softened interior pushes into a weakened area of the fibrous covering. The protruding portion of the disk then exerts pressure on a nerve root, which responds by becoming inflamed and painful. This is what is commonly referred to as a herniated, or "slipped" disc. A combination of chicory leaf and endive leaf juice can supply the body with enough magnesium-calcium-phosphorus mixture to nutritionally strengthen a "sagging" disc. The generous quantity of potassium can reduce nerve inflammation somewhat, thereby lessening the pain. Ultimately though, surgery, chiropractics, or maybe even the wearing of a back brace may become necessary for a permanent solution to the problem.

Tendinitis.   This is a condition in which the tendons become inflamed or torn. Tendons are the fibers that attach a muscle to a bone. They are usually sheathed in a membrane known as the synovium, which helps lubricate the joints and assists in smooth joint movement. Most commonly, tendinitis occurs in the shoulder, the elbow, the wrist, the thumb, the hip, the knee, and the heel. The affected area is swollen and tender, and normal movements can be limited. Athletes and people over 40 are especially susceptible to tendinitis. Besides rest and not moving the affected area too much, some therapists prescribe a high-potency mineral supplement. It is known that calcium, magnesium, and potassium are useful for reducing the swelling and tenderness associated with this temporary discomfort. Chicory and endive leaf juice contain all three of these minerals in abundance and, therefore, work to remove the problem.

METHOD OF PREPARATION

The thing to remember here is that both endive cousins need to be thoroughly washed several times in a large pan in the sink with cold tap water constantly running into it. Once this has been accomplished, remove from the pan but *don't* shake the excess water off the leaves. Just put them into your juicer wet; this gives additional liquid to make juicing easier.

If a carrot or beet is to be added for flavoring, either should be juiced separately and then mixed in with the other afterwards. Only a small amount (one-half to one cup) is necessary; too much at one time may cause bloating or intestinal gas discomfort.

CHILE PEPPERS JUICE

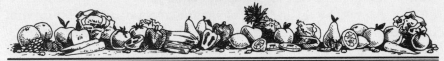

"Burning Away Fat and Relieving Pain"

DESCRIPTION

The world of chiles (*Capsicum* sp.) is both bewildering and fascinating. There are as many as 150 to 200 different varieties of chiles that have been positively identified, and there are probably still more in remote jungles of Mexico or South America that haven't been identified. New ones are being developed all the time by plant geneticists. Add to this the fact that chiles are widely spread and they cross-breed freely, and you can appreciate the impossibility of coming up with a definitive listing of chiles.

Even the spelling of the word can get confusing. *Chile* often alternates between *chili* and *chilli*. It pretty much depends, though, on how the word is being used, which part of the country you're in or even on personal whim! The general convention for proper usage is that *chile* refers to the plant or pod, while *chili* refers to the traditional dish containing meat and chiles (and sometimes beans) and *chilli* is the commercial spice powder that contains ground chiles along with a number of other spices. Then there's the country of *Chile* in South America, to add to the confusion!

Chiles share with beans (pinto, lima), maize (corn), and the cucurbits (squash, pumpkin, gourd) the distinction of being among the first plants cultivated in the Western Hemisphere. Archaeologists have found their remains in sites in both Central and South America, dating back several thousand years.

A Spanish caballero by the name of El Capitán Gonzalo Fernández de Oviedo y Valdés (1478–1537) reached tropical America at Darién, Panama in 1513. He was the first to write a history of the New World and the first to document chile peppers in those regions of land claimed by Spain. His fascinating account appeared in print in 1526 in a book entitled *História general y natural de las Indias.*

In general, the smaller the chile, the greater is its thermonuclear capacity to blow your lips right off your face! The best antidotes to the volcanic properties of chiles are dairy products such as milk, half-and-half, whipping cream, yogurt, or even ice cream. Starchy foods like bread or rice will neutralize the natural alkaloids in chiles.

The most potent chemical that can make a real fire-breathing dragon out of even the dullest personality is known as capsaicin. It survives both cooking and freezing processes to unleash its fiery sensation when least expected. The amount of capsaicin present in a chile determines its fieriness. In addition to setting off all the fire alarms within your system, this substance triggers the brain to produce endorphins, natural painkillers that promote a sense of well-being and stimulation.

In a way, consuming the more potent chiles is a form of "culinary sadomasochism" in that a certain pleasure is derived from eating something that can inflict a lot of pain on various parts of the body. Not all chiles listed here, however, will do that. Some, in fact, add a distinctive sweet flavor to whatever they're included in.

Having looked through a few other juice books on the market, I believe I can say with absolute proof that *none* of them discuss the use of chile juice per se. I don't think it's so much deliberate omission, as it is the simple lack of never having explored their full juice potential as I have done.

Bell Pepper (Green and Red).   These particular chiles have zero heat and actually have a mild sweetness to them. Both are thick-fleshed with inside seed pods. The first one is bright medium green, shaped like a cube but rounded at the edges, and sometimes tapers slightly from broad shoulders. It measures about four to five inches in length and three to four inches in diameter. It is often stuffed or used in salads and casseroles. The other is bright red, usually shaped like the green bell pepper, measures about four to five inches long and three to four inches in diameter. It is sweeter than the green bell, with crisp, fruity tones similar to ripened tomatoes. It is a favorite in salads, stews, and with pastas. Both are terrific for juicing, seed pods and all!

Habanero.   The habanero (meaning, quite literally, "from Havana" where it was probably first discovered) is dark green to orange, orange-red or red when fully ripe. It is lantern-shaped and measures about two inches long and one and one-fourth to one and one-half inches in diameter. Don't be fooled by its candy colors; there is *nothing* innocent about its looks! The ripe habanero is 30 to 50 times hotter than the jalapeño and—no fooling—can put your mouth, throat, and sinuses into the hospital Intensive Care Unit if you're not careful to use only a tiny amount. Surprisingly enough, a sliver of habanero has a wonderful, distinctive flavor with tropical fruit tones that mix well with food containing tropical fruits or tomatoes. A smidgen of fresh habanero juice in papaya, mango, pineapple or passion fruit juices is just enough to sing the chorus line from the Broadway musical hit "Hello Dolly!" in your gastrointestinal tract to get things moving in a positive direction.

Jalapeño (Green and Red).   This chile is named after the town of Jalapa in the Mexican state of Vera Cruz. It is bright medium to dark green in its unripened state, tapers to a rounded end and measures about two to three inches long and one to one and one-half inches in diameter. It is thick-fleshed and has a green vegetable flavor. It's probably the best known and most widely consumed hot chile in America, as well as the first chile ever to be taken into space in 1982. The ripe form of the green jalapeño is red and has a sweeter flavor than the green, although both hit the heat scale at 5.5. For the timid and truly reluctant who are afraid to try a few drops of habanero juice in their regular vegetable or tropical fruit juices, this is the next best thing to culinary sky diving.

Pimento.   This chile is scarlet, almost heart shaped, tapers to a point and measures about four inches long and up to three inches in diameter. It is fleshy and wonderfully sweet and aromatic and varies in strength from very mild to slightly hot. It is most commonly used in its powdered form called paprika, the best of which is still imported from Hungary. Visit the gourmet section of your supermarket or in shops that specialize in imported food items to get it. Include one or two strips with bell pepper juice for an unforgettable drinking experience.

Tabasco.   This final chile entry is bright orange-red and measures about one to one and one-half inches long and one-fourth to one-half inches in diameter. It is thin-fleshed and has a sharp, biting heat with some stemminess and hints of celery and green onion. It is used almost exclusively in the famous McIlhenny Tabasco pepper sauce. A short, quick shake of its bottled contents in bell pepper, carrot, tomato or V-8® or dark liquid chlorophyll will accelerate the chile's dynamic properties past the posted speed limit signs of moderation.

NUTRITIONAL DATA

One bell pepper (either green or red) contains about: 15 mg. calcium, 36 mg. phosphorus, 1.1 mg. iron, 21 mg. sodium, 349 mg. potassium, 690 I.U. vitamin A, 210 mg. vitamin C, and approximately 104 mg. magnesium.

The habanero and jalapeño are very high in vitamins A, C, and P or bioflavonoids. They are also good sources of potassium, folic acid, and vitamin E. Where these little firecrackers *really* shine is in two minerals, namely copper and phosphorus. Their tiny seeds are *incredibly rich* in both, which accounts for their blowtorch effects when appearing together to form capsaicin. This colorless irritant phenolic amide, in turn, triggers an escalation in the body's own "fat thermostat" setting. So when spontaneous combustion sets in, stored fat in muscle tissue begins to slowly dissolve or break up.

Numerous reports in the medical and scientific literature for the last several decades have shown that the copper-phosphorus sustained capsaicin stops all joint pain by simply anaesthetizing nerve endings so they don't produce any more "substance P" (a neurotransmitter) which conveys pain signals to the brain. A number of pain-relieving roll-on liniments and finger-applied salves that are brisk sellers right now in the health food market, all contain varying amounts of capsaicin as their primary ingredient.

The nutritional analysis for pimentos has always been for a small jar or can rather than an individual strip. The nutrients are as follows for such: 8 mg. calcium, 19 mg. phosphorus, 1.7 mg. iron, 2,600 I.U. vitamin A, and 107 mg. vitamin C. There are also trace amounts of some B-complex vitamins, vitamin E, and magnesium.

The folks on Avery Island at the southern tip of Louisiana, who manufacture the sauce named after the tabasco pepper, stated that the research they've done on it indicates high yields of vitamins A, C, and P, and minerals like copper, phosphorus, potassium, and sulphur, while only moderate amounts of vitamins B-complex and E, and calcium, magnesium, iron, and sodium appear.

THERAPEUTIC BENEFITS

Bill and Denise Smith of Wichita Falls, Kansas shared a serious medical problem between them a few years ago — the disease of obesity! With the unattractive physical shapes which accompanied it, they also experienced periodic pains in their abdomens, muscles, and joints. "We don't know if it was gout or a touch of arthritis that we had," Denise told me, "but we figured we hurt because we were so F-A-T!"

They listened to a local talk radio show I did by telephone from my home in Salt Lake City. They were especially intrigued with my short discussion on the advantages which chile peppers offered in helping people to lose weight and keep it off *permanently*, and relieving some of their aches and pains. They wrote for more information. In the series of correspondence which eventually flowed between us, I learned in detail of their "battles with the bulge" and their endurance of pain.

I put them on a simple program involving both types of bell pepper and pimento juices combined with a little carrot juice one day and a little tomato or V-8® juice the next. I had them add a quick shake of Tabasco sauce to every full glass of juice mix they drank each day with a meal. I also had them season their food regularly with granulated kelp (a seaweed) in place of black pepper, for its iodine content to stimulate the thyroid gland (an important thing to remember doing when attempting to lose weight). They also used powdered cayenne pepper in very limited amounts as an additional seasoning agent to certain foods. Ordinary table salt and black pepper were completely removed from their diets, as I don't feel either of these are very healthy to be using.

Within a matter of weeks, they started noticing a reduction, albeit small, in their waistlines and calve and buttock sizes. When they started to complain of a strong craving for sweets, I alternated their vegetable juices with tropical fruit juices every other day. This kept their "sweet tooths" satisfied; but so as not to lose the combustion action then in progress on the remainder of their fat, I instructed them to juice mere slivers of the habanero or its half-pint cousin, the jalapeño in with their tropical fruit juices. They were encouraged to wear rubber gloves when working with these atom bomb peppers so as not to injure their skin.

In the meantime they pursued a more reasonable coarse in their eating habits, although I encouraged them to snack frequently throughout the day on fresh vegetables, seeds, plain popcorn, nuts, berries, and grapes. In fact, they soon got into a regular pattern of eating more often than they had done before the program, but it was spread out into numerous snacks instead of several big meals a day. They did virtually no exercise that I know of except some limited walking.

Within five months on this program, both had lost inches off their waists, hips, thighs, buttocks, and bellies. They had more energy, were finally free of most pain, and felt better than they had in years. While the program I put them on isn't going to produce immediate results overnight or even in a week's time, it will, with patience and determination, eventually pay off handsomely for those who "stay the course."

I might also add here that the oleoresin capsaicin in chiles has been used in some nonlethal self-defense sprays for repelling criminals and, believe it or not, *bears* in Montana's Yellowstone Park and up in Alaska! In both instances, when humans and bears were hit directly in the eyes with the stuff, they turned in frenzy and ran away half-blind! Various reports of this have routinely appeared in *Chile Pepper* magazine.

AIDS   Many forms of therapy have been tried by doctors in dealing with the pervasive epidemic of acquired immune deficiency syndrome. However, not all of them have worked. And the few which have, generally have been of short-term duration at best. One AIDS survivor of five years took a very different approach to the problem. After finding that conventional medicine offered little hope, he turned his attention to hot, ethnic foods loaded with chile peppers. He wrote: "About every two days, I eat very spicy food from one of many countries that use hot spices, such as Mexico, Brazil, Burma, China (Szechuan/Hunan), Thailand, and Korea. Each cuisine is based upon the local spices, which are different, and seem to affect different micro-organisms in different ways. The most dramatic effect is from the Korean spicy pickled cabbage called *kim-chi*, which has a lot of red cayenne pepper. . . I have discovered, to my surprise, that most of the long-term survivors I know are also eating spicy food, and particularly the Korean *kim-chi*, at least once per week." And what were the final results of his daring dietary experimentation with chiles? "Four years ago, I looked like grim death, and several of my neighbors were asking my landlord if they could have my apartment, if and when . . . Since then, I gained ten pounds, and I have maintained the increased weight for well over a year. . . Frequently, people are complimenting me on how well I look—the same people who thought I was dying a few years ago. They tell me, in confidential tones, that a few years ago, they thought I had AIDS, but since my condition always seems to be improving, they know it couldn't be AIDS." His incredible story appeared in the *Journal of Orthomolecular Medicine* (5:1:25-31, 1990) under the opera pseudonym of Calaph Timmerson. The chiles apparently enhance the production of killer T-cells, interleukin-2, and other powerful immune defenses, which effectively destroy most of the AIDS virus.

Thrombosis. This is a formation of a clot within a blood vessel which can cause infarction of tissues supplied by the vessel. Studies conducted by scientists in countries which have low incidence of thrombosis, most notably Thailand and Mexico, have shown that the populations of each are heavy consumers of chile peppers. The pungent capsaicin in the peppers prevents blood cells from clumping together like grapes to produce a clot.

METHOD OF PREPARATION

Wash bell peppers with hand or liquid dish soap and then rinse thoroughly under cold tap water. Cut in halves or quarters for easier juicing. One full bell pepper (including seed pod) yields about a half cup or less of juice. For variation, try juicing a red and green one together. Then add a couple of slices of pimento and a dash of Tabasco sauce. Dilute with a half cup carrot, tomato, or V-8® juice, if necessary. Best taken after slight refrigeration.

When juicing any of the tropical fruits, such as papaya, passion fruit, pineapple, and mango, be sure to add a tiny piece the size of your small fingernail of habanero or jalapeño *during* the juicing process and *not* afterwards! Mixing a little crushed ice in with these fruit and chile juices in order to make a more smooth, milkshake-like drink is very helpful in reducing the fieriness of the peppers.

With respect to the chiles, a word ought to be said about their strong hypoglycemic properties. I never knew that peppers were so decidedly hypoglycemic until I run across an article by several Jamaican doctors which appeared in an obscure scientific publication called the *West Indian Medical Journal* (31:194–197, 1982). Mongrel dogs which were given varying amounts of the fluid extract of red pepper via a stomach tube while in an anaesthetized condition, experienced remarkably low drops in their blood sugar levels for up to several hours.

Quite amazed by this discovery, I began doing interviews with some of those whom I knew had hypoglycemia, and asked them their reactions whenever they ate Mexican or Oriental food or took cayenne pepper in capsulated form. Invariably, the majority of those questioned responded by noting that they felt some of the classic symptoms of hypoglycemia during this time: fatigue, mood swing, headache, forgetfulness, nervousness, and insomnia, among others. For this reason, those who suffer from *severe* low blood sugar, might want to rethink taking most of the chiles into their systems—the sole exceptions would be bell peppers, pimentos, and paprika.

Speaking of which, I didn't include paprika with the other chiles in "Description" for the simple reason that paprika always appears as a bright red powder made from special varieties of pepper and therefore, can't be juiced like the others. However because Hungarian paprika is very high in vitamin C and beta-carotene content, it's advisable to include a pinch in whichever of these juices you might be making.

CITRUS JUICES

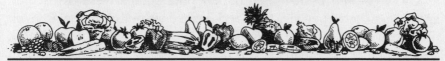

"Cranking Up the Immune System to Fight Influenza"

DESCRIPTION

Today's outstanding grapefruit (*Citrus paradisi*) is a far cry from the original one, which was called a pomelo or shaddock. While they had greater size, were puffier with thicker skins and had more seeds, they yielded very little juice and were terribly sour.

Grapefruit.   Florida, Texas, and California grow most of this nation's grapefruits. Grapefruit comes in assorted sizes and in a variety of skin and flesh colors. Some have seeds, others are seedless. The skins may be golden-yellow, red-cheeked, bronze, or russet. The flesh colors are either yellow, pink, or red. Some grapefruits are as small as a fair-sized orange, others are as big as a melon; and they come in all sizes in between. Until about fifty years ago, nearly all grapefruit were of a variety called the Duncan. They were thin-skinned, heavy, fine-flavored, and full of juice but also full of seeds.

Duncans are no longer shipped to market for table use but are grown in limited supply and sold to canneries and processors. These firms pack canned grapefruit sections and fresh or frozen concentrated grapefruit juice. The Duncans have been replaced by a seedless variety called the marsh seedless. This variety originated from a chance seedling of the Duncan variety that produced seedless grapefruit. The marsh seedless is a yellow-fleshed, seedless grapefruit that has fine flavor and texture and is fairly juicy, but it isn't quite as juicy as the Duncan. All the golden-fleshed grapefruit sold to consumers for table use are of the marsh seedless variety. Mutations of the marsh seedless have yielded fruit that have a pink- rather than a yellow-colored flesh. When darker pink strains were discovered and propagated, they yielded a red-fleshed grapefruit that was given the name of ruby red. The pinks and the reds usually command a 15-20% higher price than the yellow-fleshed grapefruit. This premium exists only because the fruit is more colorful, not because it is juicier or more flavorful. Pink, red, or yellow-fleshed fruit of comparable quality are similar in flavor and texture.

Kumquat.   Kumquat (*Fortunella margarita*) is an attractive mini-ature citrus fruit which is shaped something like an olive. It is highly prized in the Orient, where it has been cultivated for several millenniums. In the United States, it is grown on a limited scale in Florida and California.

A kumquat is quite tart and has many seeds. Its skin, like the skin of all citrus fruits, has a sharp, alcoholic flavor. Some people enjoy eating raw kumquats, skin and all, but most of those sold in North America are used for decorative purposes.

Lemon.   The lemon (*Citrus limon*) is available year-round. Most are produced in California and Florida, but Arizona brings up the lead with its share of lemon groves. Because of certain federal government regulations restricting the free flow of California lemons to the rest of the nation, we sometimes end up buying imported lemons from Spain, Italy, and Chile.

While there are several varieties of lemons, and they sometimes come from different areas, they aren't identified by variety or source at supermarkets. The high quality California lemons are packed and marketed through a co-op—Sunkist Growers, Inc., and bears their stamped logo on each one. Lemons which don't quite match these standards of excellence get to market unstamped.

The quality of a lemon is judged by the color, clearness, and texture of the skin, not by the size of the fruit. As lemons age, the light yellow color turns to a darker yellow. Lemons with scars or blemishes on their outer skins don't pass as Number Ones. The color and the clearness of the skin is no clue to its juice content even though those with blemished skins sell at lower prices at the wholesale (but not retail) level. However, the skin texture is all-important. The thinner the skin of the lemon (as well as any other citrus fruit), the higher the juice content. The smaller- and medium-sized lemons are usually thinner-skinned than the larger sized fruit. The larger lemons are always more costly by weight than the smaller ones. As a rule, the less costly, smaller lemons are a better buy. Gently rolling a hard lemon on a table with the open palm of your hand will result in a much greater juice yield.

Lime. The lime (*Citrus aurantifolia*), as with the lemon, is available year-round. Most of our limes come from Florida, but some are grown in California, while others are imported from the Yucatan in Mexico and Venezuela. Most limes are either of the Tahitian variety or the Mexican variety.

Limes are similar in flavor and texture to lemons. While they are not quite as tart, they are more fragrant than their yellow cousins. Since they are so very similar, in almost any recipe that calls for lemons, limes can be substituted, and vice versa. However, I've noticed that limes give a more subtle flavor to certain dishes than lemons do. For instance, throughout the Yucatan, a special chicken soup is always made with fresh squeezed lime juice but never lemon juice.

This ability to substitute is important for consumers to know because sometimes there is a huge difference in the prices of limes and lemons. As a rule, limes are dirt cheap in the summer months, when lemons are very costly; so don't hesitate to use limes in place of them. In the winter months, just the opposite is true, and lemons are more affordable than limes.

Limes are at their best when used to flavor beverages. They are also excellent for use on seafood, salad greens, and avocados. The fresher the lime, the darker green the skin color will be. A yellowish lime isn't too fresh and will lack the necessary acidity that gives it flavor. As a lime ages even further, the skin will show brown, scalded areas. A yellow or even a scalded lime can still be used as long as it is firm but won't be as good as a dark green lime and will be available at a much cheaper price.

Oranges

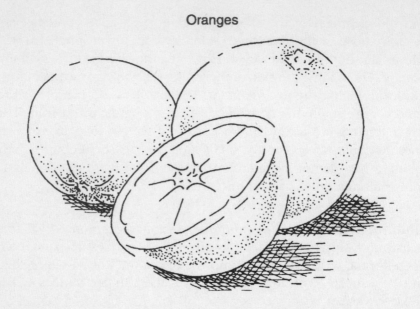

Orange.   The United States is fortunate enough to be blessed with the world's finest oranges (*Citrus sinensis*). They date back to when California and Florida belonged to Spain and orange trees were planted alongside numerous Spanish missions.

Due to differences in soil and climate, there are differences in the color, texture, and juice content of California and Florida oranges. Even when both areas grow an identical variety, the end product is not the same. Florida oranges are thinner-skinned and have more juice than the ones grown in California, but they are more difficult to peel and segment. As a rule, the Florida orange is better for squeezing into juice and the California orange is better for table use. Much of the Florida crop is used to make frozen concentrate or sold as fresh orange juice in paperboard containers and bottles.

The California oranges aren't quite as juicy and are not nearly as thin-skinned as the Florida oranges. Both the skin and the flesh of the California oranges are a deeper orange in color. All the California oranges and most of the Florida oranges are seedless, but one important Florida variety, the pineapple orange, has lots of seeds.

Both California and Florida have two major crops of oranges each year. The early crop from Florida has two varieties: the Hamlins and the pineapple oranges. The late Florida crop also has two varieties: the valencias and the pope summers. The early California crop is of the valencia variety and the late crop is known as the navel orange. Areas of Arizona that border California produce some oranges, and Texas, a major producer of grapefruit, grows a limited amount of oranges.

Tangerine. The tangerine (*Citrus reticulata*) is the best-known of the mandarins, a large group of orange-skinned varieties of citrus fruits grown throughout the Orient. The tangerine was first propagated as far back as 2000 B.C. Most tangerines we find in the supermarket produce section today are grown in the coastal state of Florida. Some are imported from Mexico before the Florida fruit is ready to harvest, but the quality of this import is nothing to write home about. The most common varieties of Florida tangerines are the Robinson and the Dancy. Both are similar in texture, flavor, and color, although the Robinsons attain a larger size. Tangerines are not identified by variety at the supermarket fruit stands.

Tangerines arrive in October and are out of season in February. The early arrivals are often a trifle too tart, and those at the very tail end of the season tend to be lacking in sufficient juice. Florida tangerines are in their prime during the month of December. This is the best time to buy them for juicing purposes. It should be noted here that another type of mandarin, called the honey tangerine, is firmer and juicier than the regular tangerine but more difficult to peel and segment and has a fair amount of seeds. However, if you can find it and get past these few obstacles, you'll find its flesh is very sweet and has a rich, deep orange color.

Ugli Fruit. The name given to ugli fruit (*Citrus* sp.) is quite appropriate. This has got to be the sorriest, saddest, most disgusting-looking variety of the citrus fruits I believe I've ever laid eyes on. It looks like a crummy grapefruit with a rough, loose-fitting, thick skin. The dull skin color is a mixture of green and russet-yellow. When fully ripe, the yellow portion of the skin takes on an orange-colored tint. The fruit feels spongy and the fruit comes to a point at the stem end. However, in spite of its hideous-looking, elephant hidelike peel, a surprisingly flavorful, juicy, sweet, fine-textured, pink-tinted flesh lurks beneath.

Ugli fruit is native to the island of Jamaica in the Caribbean Sea. It is probably an offshoot of the combination of a pomelo (the original grapefruit) and a sweet or mandarin orange. The Jamaican crop isn't very big, and since the supply is very limited, prices are always on the expensive side. Attempts to grow ugli fruit in Florida have not met with much success. One citrus grower gave his own opinion why it doesn't do well there; "We have so much beauty in our state, there just isn't any place for ugli-ness."

But for all of the gaffes and guffaws this mean-looking citrus draws from many skeptics, I've discovered it to be quite a nice-flavored fruit, maybe even a tad sweeter than your ruby red grapefruit. Interestingly enough, while many middle-class and low-income people shun it, due to lack of understanding and appreciation of just how good it tastes, a fair amount of well-to-do folks, who can afford it, buy ugli fruit for something different and out of the ordinary. In doing so, they soon find out, as I did, that in spite of its odd name and shabby appearance, there is a very delicious juice inside just waiting to be squeezed out and slowly savored like a good bottle of vintage wine.

NUTRITIONAL DATA

One large grapefruit contains: 51 mg. calcium, 51 mg. phosphorus, 1.3 mg. iron, 3 mg. sodium, 434 mg. potassium, 30 I.U. vitamin A, some B-complex vitamins, and 122 mg. vitamin C. The inside white rind of the grapefruit peel contains considerable bioflavonoids, especially hesperidin and rutin, which are necessary for the maintenance of the small blood capillaries. These bioflavonoids also help to set the body's "fat thermostat" higher in order to chemically "burn" away excess stored fat.

One kumquat yields: 12 mg. calcium, 4 mg. phosphorus, 0.1 mg. iron, 1 mg. sodium, 44 mg. potassium, 110 I.U. vitamin A, traces of some B-complex vitamins, and 7 mg. vitamin C. Kumquats also contain small amounts of magnesium, manganese, chromium and zinc—trace elements which are useful in treating certain autoimmune disorders such as arthritis, lupus, and Crohn's disease.

One tablespoon of raw lemon juice has: 1 mg. calcium, 2 mg. phosphorus, 21 mg. potassium, 7 mg. vitamin C, and trace amounts of magnesium, iron, sodium, vitamin A, and some of the B-complex vitamins. Lemon juice also contains very small amounts of trace elements like tin, zinc, vanadium, and molybdenum.

In one tablespoon of raw lime juice you'll find: 1 mg. calcium, 2 mg. phosphorus, 16 mg. potassium, 5 mg. vitamin C, and trace amounts of iron, sodium, vitamin A, and some of the B-complex vitamins and even lesser amounts of germanium, tin, selenium, and zinc.

One cup of freshly squeezed orange juice contains: 27 mg. calcium, 42 mg. phosphorus, 0.5 mg. iron, 2 mg. sodium, 400 mg. potassium, 500 I.U. vitamin A, 1 mg. niacin, trace amounts of other B-complex vitamins and 124 mg. vitamin C. Orange juice also has an undetermined amount of boron in it.

One cup of freshly squeezed tangerine juice contains: 44 mg. calcium, 35 mg. phosphorus, 0.5 mg. iron, 2 mg. sodium, 440 mg. potassium, 1,040 I.U. vitamin A, some B-complex vitamins, and 77 mg. vitamin C. Of all the citrus fruits, tangerines seem to have a little more silicon than the others do.

Ugli fruit is quite high in potassium, phosphorus, vitamins A, C, and P (bioflavonoids), with moderate amounts of calcium, some B-complex vitamins, and magnesium, and marginal amounts of manganese, chromium, and zinc. This is the only citrus fruit I know of which has a trace amount of iodine in it, too.

THERAPEUTIC BENEFITS

According to the authors of the book, *Islands, Plants, and Polynesians: An Introduction to Polynesian Ethnobotany* (Portland: Dioscorides Press, 1991) the original grapefruit, called pomelo or shaddock, grows in great abundance throughout the jungles of Malaysia and Indonesia and as far east as Fiji and Tonga. In all of these tropical forest areas, the fruit is peeled and pounded with mallets in large wooden bowls for its juice to reduce fevers incurred from malaria and dysentery.

Vu Thi Thuoc is a young nurse in her early thirties, residing in the Vietnamese city of Hue, near the Gulf of Tonkin. When she speaks in the peculiar accent of her native tongue, she does so in a soft, drawling, almost inaudible way. Early on in a conversation several summers ago, she used the expression "de thuong" to describe me. Only after it was translated for my benefit could I begin to appreciate the high compliment just paid to me. She had told me I was "very likeable and charming." In attempting to tell her that she was also "de thuong," I got my pronunciation of the second word a little mixed up and ended up saying something else with a totally different meaning to it. We enjoyed a good-natured laugh over my mistake.

I was in that part of Asia again to gather some additional material on folk healing for other book projects I had in mind of doing some day. In the different remedies which Vu Thi relies upon to treat the many sick people in her care, along with some Western drugs, of course, there is kumquat juice. She said that it is the best thing she knows of for treating all types of lung problems, including bronchitis and pneumonia.

Remembering this piece of advice sometime later when back in the States, I recommended kumquats to a California man who was having a hard time shaking the flu, which by now was turning into pneumonia he feared. He started taking the juice each day according to my instructions—one cup in the morning on an empty stomach—and within eleven days he reported a surprising turnabout in his lingering illness.

I've discovered that the worst case of badly infected sore throat can be easily cured with two simple solutions. The first is to put a pinch of ordinary table salt into one-fourth cup of freshly squeezed lemon juice. (The lemon juice available from supermarkets in the yellow plastic squeeze container shaped like a lemon will do as a reasonable substitute if you don't want to go to the trouble all the time of cutting and squeezing fresh lemon.)

Then slowly gargle with small sips of this juice for about one minute before swallowing. It will burn like Hades, of course, in the beginning, but the pain will gradually diminish as the throat becomes accustomed to this treatment. The entire gargling procedure with the amount recommended should take about three minutes or so.

The next course of action to take is to tilt the head as far back as you can and open the mouth wide. Insert the plastic dispenser end of 60 percent bee propolis from Montana Naturals and squeeze just enough of this brown, bitter, sticky solution to the back of the throat. It will feel as if you're dripping hot candle wax back there. There will be an almost instant reaction of burning, which will be followed immediately by a sealing sensation as the bee glue solidifies and covers the inflamed mucus tissue it has just been applied on.

You'll be able to swallow much easier after this, though it isn't recommended you drink anything more until the next morning. By that time, your throat will have become healed enough that swallowing will no longer be a difficult thing to do.

Lime juice diluted with a little warm water and slowly sipped will help to relieve muscle aches and cramps accompanying even the most stubborn influenza. Figure on taking two tablespoonfuls per half cup warm water every three to four hours on an empty stomach. A more delicious alternative to this is to make some hot chicken soup with part of an old stewing hen, garlic, onion, celery, potato, parsley, and four whole limes, peeled and quartered in enough water to cover. Cook on medium heat for one and one-half hours, or you can squeeze the juice from these four limes and add to this soup about fifteen minutes before it's done.

Many people resort to canned or bottled orange juice to drink when they're sick with the common cold or influenza. The problem, though, is that the pasturization process depletes some of the meager vitamin C contents. So it's advisable to drink only freshly squeezed orange juice but at *room temperature* and not chilled or cold! The body will be able to accept it a lot better if it's not iced or too cool.

A Prized Congestion Fighter. In the summer of 1980, I went to the People's Republic of China with a group of 31 medical students and three other faculty advisors as part of an American Medical Students' Association-sponsored trip. We toured many different cities and saw quite a bit of the healing arts while there. I remember learning from the Soochow Chinese Traditional Medical Hospital in the city of Soochow, near Shanghai, that *ch'ing p'i* or tangerine juice was wonderful for breaking up mucus congestion in the throat, sinuses, lungs, and stomach. It also helps to clear the liver and alleviate body aches and pain due to various strains of influenza.

Ugli fruit juice is employed in such places as Jamaica, the Cayman Islands, the Turks and Caicos Islands, and Haiti for indigestion, abdominal cramps, nausea, and vomiting due to "stomach flu." Where food cannot easily be kept down due to different types of intestinal infections, this has seemed to serve as an old reliable standby.

One of the much touted nutrients in citrus fruits has been vitamin C. This vitamin has been extensively studied by two time

Nobel laureate Dr. Linus Pauling. In a conversation with Dr. Pauling, who as of this writing in the summer of 1993 was already into his nineties, I learned something which is fairly common knowledge among many of his colleagues but not too well known by the general public at large. For over a decade now, he has successfully *held in abeyance* his own cancer of the prostate gland, which has claimed other less fortunate ones than himself.

Dr. Pauling, of course, has taken megadoses of this vitamin for years in allottments well exceeding 100,000 milligrams; but I found it interesting to hear that he also drinks ample amounts of freshly squeezed citrus juices every day for breakfast, which gives him the same vitamin, only in a fresher form.

Sexually Transmissible Diseases. The most common sexually transmissible disease (STD) in the U.S. is chlamydia, which affects about 4 million young adults each year. The parasitic microorganisms that cause it are Chlamydia trachomatis and Chlamydia psittaci. Such organisms are larger than viruses but smaller than bacteria. Syphilis is another STD, caused by the bacterium Treponema pallidum. Historians think this is what Native Americans gave to the Europeans when they first came to the Western Hemisphere. Gonorrhea is a third type of STD and is pervasive throughout the world. An estimated 250 million people are infected with it each year. Gonorrhea is caused by a bacterium called Neisseria gonorrhea, which many people carry without developing signs of illness. The parasites or bacteria responsible for these and other STDs share one thing in common: they fare very poorly in the presence of ascorbic acid. Vitamin C shuts down their abilities to obtain nourishment from the blood supplies they're swimming in. Furthermore, ascorbic acid "poisons" the blood they depend on for their existence. Vitamin C also enhances immune defenses, which can then go after these microorganisms and effectively kill them. Ascorbic acid also neutralizes the purulent matter resulting from such infectious diseases, so that further damage isn't done to the body. All citrus fruits are very rich in vitamin C content.

Staph Infection. Staphylococcus is a genus of Gram-positive bacteria. S. pyogenes aureus is the common species causing what we know as staph infection, food poisoning, pneumonia, osteomyelitis, endocarditis, and other infections. Their metabolic behavior is respiratory and fermentative. Ascorbic acid, however, denies them their cellular breathing ability, and reverses the acid sour environment they thrive in. Citrus juices are teeming with plenty of vitamin C.

Tonsillitis.   This is an acute inflammation or infection of the tonsils. The invasion of streptococcus, a Gram-positive genus of bacteria, is one of the most common causes of this condition. Ascorbic acid attacks the species S. pyogenes in the mouth, throat, and lungs where it resides. Vitamin C also stimulates the immune system to produce more macrophages or scavenger cells, which literally gobble up strept bacteria. Citrus juices are rich in vitamin C and good for gargling and drinking in such cases.

METHOD OF PREPARATION

Each of the citrus fruits mentioned here needs to be peeled before getting juiced. In doing so, care should be taken *not* to remove the slightly bitter white membrane next to the peel. In fact, if anything, it should be scraped from the inside peel with a sharp paring knife and included with the rest of the fruit when juicing. Therein lies much nutritional goodness in the form of bioflavonoids.

The more sour citrus fruits should be used on a limited scale and only in small amounts due to their excess hyperacidity. Common sense will need to be relied upon here, because not everyone's digestive tract will be able to tolerate very much of such acidic juices. This is especially so for older people. It might be helpful to combine some of these sour juices in with more flavorful citrus juices. For instance, one part lime juice to five parts orange or tangerine juice makes a delightful and healthful drink.

The juice should be strained through a coarse wire strainer of some kind to catch any seeds that come through the juicing process. For some reason, kumquat juice goes better with something bland like pear juice than it does with the other citrus fruits.

CUCUMBER JUICE

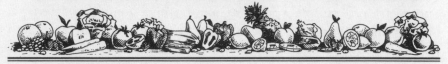

"Best Skin Toner Around"

DESCRIPTION

Cucumber (*Cucumis sativus*) is related closely to squash and melons. It is produced in all states and available year-round. During the winter months, supplies from California, Florida, and Texas are supplemented by imports from Mexico and the islands of the West Indies.

There are many varieties of cucumbers, but they can be broken down into three basic types: the run-of-the-mill, smooth-skinned garden cucumbers; the small, warty-skinned pickles; and the elongated, almost seedless European cucumbers.

The best-flavored cucumber, but not necessarily the most handsome in the crowd, is a pickle (also called a Kirby). The Kirby is a variety that is pale green and off-white in color. It is quite small, but the smaller the better. It isn't very symmetrical and the skin is warty. However, in this case looks can be quite deceiving to say the least! The Kirby is crisp, crunchy, and the tiny seeds give them a fine flavor. The Kirby is used to make the dill pickles that you buy in jars in supermarkets.

The smallest variety of pickle is called the gherkin. It is also very tasty when consumed raw, but seldom ever found in supermarkets. Commercial processors contract for them by the ton and pay growers a whopping amount of money.

When choosing any type of cucumber, the darker the color (except for the Kirby), the better. A yellow color indicates old age and possibly hard seeds. The slim medium or small cukes are preferable to the big fat ones. By all means, avoid any cukes that are puffy, soft, withered, or shriveled (soft ones sometimes have a nasty taste to them). Cucumbers keep for more than a week in the refrigerator, but it is preferable to use them in a couple of days after purchase.

NUTRITIONAL DATA

One cup of raw, unpared, sliced cucumbers yields the following amount of nutrients: 26 mg. calcium, 28 mg. phosphorus, 1.2 mg. iron, 6 mg. sodium, 168 mg. potassium, 260 I.U. vitamin A, trace amounts of some B-complex vitamins (such as thiamin, riboflavin and niacin), 12 mg. vitamin C, and 13 mg. magnesium. It also has traces of boron and chlorine in it.

THERAPEUTIC BENEFITS

Paul Bragg, who died some time ago in advanced years, was a very popular health speaker and writer as far back as 1935, when the medical and scientific communities were a lot less inclined to accept alternative ways as they are now. In an article he had published in an old issue of *Nature's Path*, he said this about cucumber juice: "There is nothing more nourishing for the skin to have than the liquid juice from the cucumber. The nutrition-rich water that it contains, when taken into the body, adds lustre to the hair, sparkle to the eye, color to the lips, tone to the skin, and spring to the step."

Mr. Bragg considered it to be one of nature's finest "liquid rejuvenators for keeping someone feeling and *looking* youthful and radiant. He insisted that the liquid nourishment provided from the juice, "flushes the system out in a most wonderful and, if I may say so, daring way." He never qualified what he meant by that last statement of "daring way." But it suffices to say that when the *entire* cuke is juiced, peel and all, it sets into motion a unique cleansing action within the body that liberally removes accumulated pockets of old waste material and chemical toxins. Once these are out of the body, he wrote, "then you are on your way to glowing health again!"

It is said that Mr. Bragg, for whom cucumber was an important mainstay of his daily juice routine, didn't have very many wrinkles in his skin because of this, even though he was out in the sun a lot due to his love of swimming and other outdoor physical activities. Some think the natural oils present in the peel may have something to do with how resilient and remarkably clear the skin can look following a lengthy period of cucumber juicing.

Also try this technique the next time you're bothered with roaches and ants. Soak strips of cucumber peel in the juice for an hour. Then remove and dry them in a 200-degree oven until quite brittle. Next run them through your food blender with a couple of bay leaves that have also been soaked in the same cucumber juice and then permitted to dry. Spread the resulting powder along baseboards and cupboards. Reapply every one and one-half weeks.

Insect Stings.   A mother in Alabama told me once how she treated a bee sting on the bottom of her young daughter's foot, after the girl had accidentally stepped on a bee. "I went over to where my cucumbers were growing, picked one off the vine, took it inside, peeled and coarsely cut part of it, then pureed it in my food blender. After this, I poured the thick mixture into the bottom of an empty plastic bread sack and then had my girl stick her foot into this. She kept it there for about an hour or until all of the throbbing pain, swelling and itching had ceased."

Poison Ivy/Poison Oak/Poison Sumac Rash.   These three plants produce a severe, itchy rash when they come in contact with the skin. A rash can develop after touching clothing, equipment, or animals that have brushed against them. Even burning their leaves releases chemicals into the air that can cause rashes and, more seriously, lung inflammation if the fumes are inhaled. The allergens present in the plants' sap provoke a skin reaction by activating defensive mechanisms in the immune system. Antibodies form, leading to the release of other body chemicals that produce the characteristic rash and itchiness. The nutrient-rich moisture in cucumber, when applied to the surface of the skin, immediately puts out the "fire" caused by this trio of plant saps. When the juice is taken internally, the potassium salts work to stop further production of the antibodies responsible for the external irritations.

Sunburn. Proper procedures for treating sunburn call for *cool* baths or showers and the application of *cool* compresses to the skin to alleviate pain, *not* ice or ice water! In more severe cases, the intake of fluids is necessary to prevent dehydration. Also blisters should *not* be broken. The moisture rich contents of cucumber meets all of these requirements. It is cooling, but not chilling. There is enough fluid in cucumber to prevent dehydration, and cucumber will prevent blisters from suddenly erupting. It is the *ultimate* sunburn treatment!

METHOD OF PREPARATION

Two medium-sized cucumbers should yield close to one and one-half cups of juice. First, wash both cukes with soap and water, then rinse under the sink tap, after which, they should be dried off with a towel. These precautionary measures are necessary to remove some of the wax which the produce industry applies before they reach your supermarket.

A nice addition to cucumber juice is one-fourth cup parsley or alfalfa juice, flavored with an equal amount of fresh carrot or beet juice. These help to expel uric acid from the system more quickly.

DANDELION JUICE

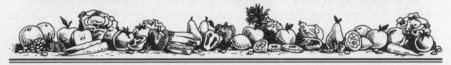

"Rescuing the Liver from Dietary Abuse"

DESCRIPTION

Dandelions (*Taraxacum officinale*) are so abundant and familiar that they hardly need description. The name dandelion is a corruption of the French *dents de lion*, referring to the jagged-toothed leaves that can be said to resemble a lion's well-equipped jaw. The bright yellow blossoms are very sensitive to light and weather conditions, closing up before darkness and storms. When the flower head has matured, it closes again with the calyx drawn in a cylindrical shape around the ripening ovaries. When the seeds inside have ripened, it reopens to form the familiar flubby ball of seeds; each with its own "parachute" waiting to be dispersed by a breeze.

In practical application, it is for spring greens that the dandelions are most well known. In early spring, before much of the plant world is stirring, the leaves of the dandelion are at their prime for eating. It seems that after the plant blossoms, its leaves become tough, bitter, and less desirable as a food or for juicing purposes. But if some apple cider vinegar is used in any salad containing *older* dandelion leaves or in the juice of mature leaves, the tartness of the vinegar itself does wonders in cutting down the sharp bitterness of the greens.

There is a very efficient technique for collecting dandelion greens. Use a butcher knife, old hunting knife, or small machete when out gathering them. Squat down on your haunches and slip the knife under the entire plant and slice it off at the top of the root. This permits you to gather the whole plant, including the best part, the delicate unopened center called the heart or crown.

NUTRITIONAL DATA

One hundred edible grams of dandelion leaves, which is about three and one-half ounces or nearly one-fourth pound, yields the following nutrients: 309 mg. calcium, 66 mg. phosphorus, 3.1 mg. iron, 397 mg. potassium, 14,000 I.U. vitamin A, trace amounts of some B-complex vitamins, and 35 mg. vitamin C. It is also high in magnesium.

The late Euell Gibbons, a popular naturalist, plant forager, prolific writer, and television personality during the mid-sixties and seventies, once said of this lowly lawn weed:

> "It is an excellent source of calcium and potassium, and the best known source of vitamin A among the green vegetables. And yet, we spend millions on herbicides to kill the dandelions in our lawns, while we pay millions more for diet supplements to give ourselves the vitamins and minerals that the dandelion could easily furnish."

He would occasionally throw "wild parties" for a selected group of friends. Every food and beverage served would have come from the wild, hence the name of "wild parties." He liked to tell his friends that the "green punch" they were drinking was really his special recipe for dandelion greens, pigweed, and parsley juices combined into one concoction.

He claimed that this "green punch," which he flavored with pineapple juice and Canadian Club Soda, had more iron and vitamins A and C in it than any other foods listed in the USDA Agricultural Handbook No. 8 entitled, *Composition of Foods*. He called it his "feel good, health drink!"

THERAPEUTIC BENEFITS

One would not think of the liver as a primary organ of concern in dealing with an autoimmune disease such as rheumatoid arthritis. But the late Rudolf Fritz Weiss, M.D., author of the popular German best-seller, *Lehrbuch der Phytotherapie* (Stuttgart: Hippokrates Verlag GmbH, 1985) claimed that it was "the point of action at which chronic degenerative joint disease began."

Dr. Weiss routinely recommended either dandelion tea, fluid extract, or the juice for arthritic conditions. Of these three, he felt that dandelion juice was the most helpful and effective. He prescribed for his arthritic patients that they take one-half cup of the juice morning and evening on an empty stomach. Sometimes he would vary it a little by including equal parts of dandelion and watercress juice for more severe cases in which the patients had become quite crippled and unable to move about very much.

In one unique episode, a Frau Muhlenstein, age 61, was diagnosed as having "nodose rheumatism." Her clinical symptoms bore all the earmarks of classic rheumatoid arthritis (RA): gradual swellings in the hands and feet that were symmetrical and spindle-shaped, especially in the joint areas; smooth and shiny skin; brittle and discolored nails; a "hot" sensation around each swollen joint; an irregular low fever; some weight loss; and a general ill feeling.

Other medical specialists with whom she had previously consulted had put her on various types of therapies—corticosteroids, golds salts, ibuprofen, and salicylates—which proved of little benefit. Out of desperation she turned to Dr. Weiss. Within a week, after being on the dandelion-watercress juice program and a restricted diet, she began showing improvement. Within two weeks, she began to have movement in her gnarled fingers and toes. Within three weeks, the joint swelling had substantially subsided. Within four weeks, virtually all pain was gone. And within one and one-half months, she was able to grip a pen, pot handle, door knob, fruit jar, and even shake someone else's hand without any problems. In two months, she was able to begin walking up to a mile a day, including climbing stairs again. Within three months, she was able to attend dances with her husband and enjoy her favorite waltzes.

Dr. Weiss had similar stories of success for other ailments originating from the liver and kidneys, such as obesity, gout, hypertension, arteriosclerosis/atherosclerosis, Bright's disease, and kidney stones. In fact, he attributed many of our degenerative and autoimmune disorders to a breakdown in the functions of the liver, one of the most vital organs in our bodies. Dandelion was God's very special remedy for these things, he insisted.

Dr. Weiss maintained that dandelion juice was good for a number of other conditions, not all of which were connected with dietary abuse of the liver. While he didn't feel the juice would cure any of them, he felt it could do no harm and might, in fact, actually do some good where others didn't seem to work.

Herpes Simplex. Herpes is one of the oldest known viruses to man. It has existed since the Jurassic Age of dinosaurs. As goofy as it sounds, some paleontologists think that small nodules on the thick hides of some dinosaurs may have been the result of a herpes infection of some kind. It's hard to imagine such a beast with chickenpox or shingles (both caused by this virus). What is known for sure is that herpes is a greasy-looking virus, prefers an acidic environment, and likes to hide in the ganglion or sensory nerves located just beneath the surface of the skin. Dandelion is loaded with mineral salts, which quickly alkalinize acidic blood. The enormous vitamin A content then takes over to minimize further viral activity by boosting immune defenses.

Night Blindness. A German doctor, S. Niedermeier mentioned that vitamins A and B-complex work in the liver to restore deficient dark adaptation. He also routinely prescribed a juice extract of dandelion flowers for night blindness. He attributed their remarkable success to a particular substance known as helenin, which produces more visual purple for the eye. To be effective for this, though, helenin requires the presence of a certain amount of vitamin A, he discovered. Dandelion leaf and flower, of course, are very high in this and B vitamins. Through experimentation he found that dandelion helenin is also good for improving the nyctalopia that accompanies retinitis pigmentosa. His highly interesting report appeared over four decades ago in *Deutsche medizinische Wochenschrift* (76:210, February 16, 1951).

Tuberculosis. TB is an infectious disease that was one of the leading causes of death worldwide in centuries preceding our own. For many decades it has been virtually extinct. Now with the increasing rise in poverty and homelessness, the disease is again making a strong comeback. TB is caused by a bacterium called tubercle bacillus or Mycobacterium tuberculosis. It's spread from person to person in droplets of saliva that are expelled by coughing, sneezing, speaking, or even exhaling. The droplets evaporate, and the bacilli remain airborne. TB develops when a susceptible person with weakened immune defenses inhales the bacilli. Dandelion leaf juice helps out in several different ways. First, its strong vitamin A content acts as an effective antibiotic in stopping the progress of TB. Secondly, the rich combination of calcium potassium salts chemically "strip" the bacilli from moist mucosal tissue in the lungs where they prefer to colonize. Thirdly, certain plant alcohols in the leaves (notably xanthophyll or lutein) disinfect the lungs, making it much harder for the bacilli to remain there.

METHOD OF PREPARATION

Select dandelion greens from an area that hasn't been sprayed with herbicides. Pick them wearing gloves or cut off the top part of the plant with a knife level to the ground as previously described. Rinse them in a colander to remove bugs and dirt. Then cut or tear to juicing size. You can juice fresh watercress right along with them, if you like. The younger dandelion leaves will make a sweeter juice than older leaves picked later in the summer or fall.

Drinking one cup of dandelion juice by itself or in combination with an equal amount of watercress, will give the body a "natural high" or incredible sensation of energy when the juice hits the liver. In some cases, this may be somewhat overpowering for older people or those with delicate digestive tracts. In the event this proves to be so, simply dilute the dandelion juice with a little carrot juice.

DATE-FIG JUICES

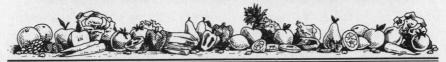

"Pleasant Stimulation for Sluggish Bowels"

DESCRIPTION

The date (*Phoenix dactylifera L.*) is the fruit of a tall palm tree known as the date palm. When young David the shepherd boy was still composing his songs and prayers unto God, he wrote this in Psalms 92:12: "The righteous shall flourish like the palm tree. . ." In ancient times, the date palm was symbolic of moral uprightness and heaven-sent prosperity.

Dates are still the staff of life for people who dwell in the arid regions of North Africa and the Middle East. The date palm bears its first fruit in the fourth year and continues to do so, with little or no care, and under far from ideal growing conditions, for the next seventy-five years.

In the United States, dates are grown commercially, on a fairly large scale, in the desert areas of California and Arizona, but some are also imported from Israel. The best-known variety is called the Deglet Noor. The largest and most costly variety is called the Medjoul. I often get specially wrapped boxes (32 dates per box) of the expensive kind ($26.98) from Red Copper of Alamo, Texas, which I refrigerate and nibble on whenever the occasion suits me. The Medjoul date is about the closest thing to a Divine Flavor that I've ever tasted!

117

Figs (*Ficus carica L.*) date back to the Garden of Eden and happens to be the second fruit recorded in the Bible when Adam and Eve made for themselves garments to hide their nakedness. (The first "Forbidden Fruit," according to Apocryphal and Talmudic references was the grape!) To sit under one's own fig tree was the Jewish concept of peace and prosperity as mentioned in I Kings 4:25. Figs are still eaten fresh or dried and threaded on long strings throughout much of Asia Minor. They are an important cash crop in Greece, Turkey, and Italy. Nearly all the figs grown commercially in America are produced in California, although Texas has an expanding crop that is usually sold to canners. Figs are also grown in many home gardens as far north as New York.

Figs are perishable and have a very limited shelf life. They are somewhat fragile and have to be picked, packed, and shipped with the utmost care. The fruit is not only delicate to handle but also has a very delicate flavor. A ripe, plump, soft fig is a real sweetmeat. Its sweetness makes it useful in pastry and cookie fillings. Fig Newtons® have almost become a standard part of the growing up process for many of us.

There are several varieties of figs and they come primarily in two colors: light (also called green or white) and dark (also called black or purple). The best known light varieties are the Calmyrnas and the Kadotas. The best known dark varieties are the Black Missions (these were first planted by Catholic monks in California)

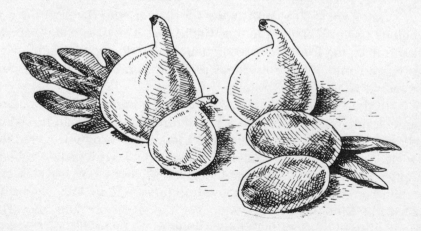

Dates and Figs

and the Brown Turkeys (named after the country and not the Thanksgiving bird).

NUTRITIONAL DATA

Ten dates yield the following nutrients: 47 mg. calcium, 50 mg. phosphorus, 2.4 mg. iron, 1 mg. sodium, 518 mg. potassium, 40 I.U. vitamin A, 1.8 mg. niacin, and very little vitamin C.

One large fig contains: 23 mg. calcium, 14 mg. phosphorus, 0.4 mg. iron, 1 mg. sodium, 126 mg. potassium, 50 I.U. vitamin A, traces of some B-complex vitamins, and 1 mg. vitamin C.

THERAPEUTIC BENEFITS

I had an interesting and somewhat unexpected experience involving dates and figs together in the summer of 1980. Our group, the American Medical Students Association was then on its way to the People's Republic of China, with temporary stopovers in Cairo, Bombay, and Addis Ababa.

Because of the enormous preparation it had taken for me to get ready for this trip—I was one of several faculty advisors to a group of medical students—everything was pretty hectic and rushed for a few days prior to my first flight to New York City to connect with our international flight that left from JFK Airport around midnight.

Now all of this stress and tension had produced a temporary situation of constipation in me. In fact, I had not had a real good bowel movement in 72 hours. During our brief layover in Egypt, I wandered along a public sidewalk not far from the airport and inspected the wares being offered by different food vendors, many of whom had set up shop on top of blankets spread out on the ground.

I was tempted by some luscious looking dates and figs, and ended up buying ten of each after the usual haggling for a "fair" price. These I put into an empty plastic sack I had brought with me and took them back onto the plane, where I carefully washed them off in one of those tiny restrooms most of us have had the misfortune of using sometime in our lives.

I leisurely ate them and thought nothing more about my constipation problem until our next longer stopover in Ethiopia.

Imagine my delight to discover the next morning the much awaited and greatly anticipated "call of nature," which I promptly and gladly responded to. That speaks well of dates and figs working in unison to stimulate a lazy or severely blocked colon.

Celiac Disease.   Also called sprue, this is usually classified as a malabsorption syndrome. Celiac disease is a chronic intestinal disorder in which intolerance to gluten—a protein found in grains—interferes with the proper absorption of many nutrients. Dates and figs contain unique protein carbohydrate complexes and mineral salts which halt an abnormal response started by gluten in the small intestine, leading to an overproduction of white blood cells. The spice cardamom also works in a similar way; therefore, it should be used in date-fig juice both as a flavoring and medicinal agent.

Insomnia.   The consumption of carbohydrate-rich foods towards bedtime will, quite often, induce sleep very soon thereafter. A little date-fig juice may be the perfect nightcap an insomniac is after, provided he or she doesn't have any blood-sugar problems.

Coughing and Whooping Cough.   I had an aging male baritone, who once sang for the Metropolitan Opera years ago, tell me at the New Life Expo in New York City in the Spring of 1993 that he always sucked and nibbled on pieces of black mission fig or pitted date (which he previously wrapped in foil) before a performance. He claimed that this helped him not to lose his voice or accidentally cough during a critical moment of deep singing. He thought it was the sugar in the juice which coated his vocal chords. I have seen honey, molasses, syrup, and sugar water used for stopping a case of whooping cough, all of which are incredibly sweet. Maybe the sugar in them and date-fig juice may act as an antispasmodic under such extreme circumstances.

Wounds.   Common white sugar has been used as a folk remedy for treating open wounds and sores in many parts of the world with very good success. Honey has also been placed into deep cavity wounds to prevent gangrene from setting in. Perhaps using date-fig juice, which is very high in sugar content, might serve an equal purpose in promoting rapid healing of such injuries. The process by which these agents work is mostly enzymatic in nature.

METHOD OF PREPARATION

Use pitted dates for easier juicing purposes. Wash some under tap water, but don't pat them dry with a towel. The extra water will make them juice better. Do the same with figs, but cut off their stems before juicing.

Because dates and figs are *incredibly sweet,* some wisdom and good judgment must be used in the amount you intend to take. In fact, it is better to dilute your date-fig concentrate with a little carrot juice. Also, *no more* than one-half cup of straight date-fig concentrate should be consumed at one time.

Those who have blood sugar problems, like diabetes and hypoglycemia, should not attempt to use these juices for constipation, simply because they're apt to produce adverse reactions.

See also Papaya-Mango Juices for related problem uses. *A cautionary note is raised here for those with blood sugar problems, allergies, or yeast infections.* Due to the high amount of natural sugars present, the use of these juices should be severely restricted under such conditions.

FENNEL JUICE

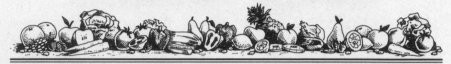

"Say Good-Bye to Heartburn"

DESCRIPTION

Fennel (*Foeniculum vulgare*) is a hardy perennial often grown as an annual. It is a large plant, standing up to six feet high, with yellow flower heads and bright green feathery leaves. It can be grown very easily in ordinary soil in a backyard of a house or else in a large pot in an apartment or condominium (provided it's set by a large window for plenty of sunlight). It will stand for several years, especially if it's not permitted to flower.

Fennel is native to southern Europe, where it has been used since time immemorial. The Romans used it a great deal and, no doubt, were responsible for introducing it into Great Britain. It was later taken to America and today in California it is one of the most common naturalized weeds. Commercially, fennel is grown for seed in many countries, particularly in France, Germany, and Italy, but also in India, Japan, and America. Indeed, there is scarcely a country outside the humid tropics where one will not find fennel being grown.

The flavor of fennel varies greatly according to the type. Wild fennel is slightly bitter and has no anise flavor. Sweet (or Roman) fennel, on the other hand, lacks the bitter principle and tastes strongly of anise. In fact, it contains large quantities of the essential oil, anethole, which makes up 90 percent of the essential oil in anise itself. Bitter fennel is the type most cultivated in central Europe and Russia, while the sweet fennel is the type usually grown in Italy,

France, and Greece. It makes quite a difference which type is used for flavoring or juicing.

The best time to drink a little fennel juice is when you're eating any kind of seafood, pork, veal, Italian cooking, French cuisine, or anything else which is heavy in fat, sugar, spices, or sauces. All one needs, actually, is just very small occasional sips from one-fourth cup fennel juice to help a huge meal digest a lot easier.

NUTRITIONAL DATA

A quarter cup of fresh fennel juice contains moderate-to-high amounts of calcium, magnesium, potassium, and phosphorus, with lesser amounts of iron, zinc, manganese, vitamin A, and some of the B-complex vitamins.

THERAPEUTIC BENEFITS

Vic Jones, a New Orleans jazz musician thinks he has found the "perfect answer" to heart burn and acid indigestion. "All this Creole and Cajun food we love to pack away down here in Orleans," he said in his typical bayou drawl, "tends to make us feel as if we're gonna split our sides like a stuck pig! Man, some of those spicy dishes really get to me sometimes," he added, while patting his substantial stomach girth and pulling a face of mock pain.

He told me in the fall of 1992, while I was passing through there, that "little sips of fennel juice does the trick every time in relieving me of my eating miseries." He claimed that it had never failed to work for anyone else to whom it had been heartily recommended.

Another "big feller" I know down Texas way, "Duke" Smith found relief from his many cases of heart burn, acid indigestion, hiatal hernia, diarrhea, and intestinal gas with the same remedy, but only after I had personally recommended it based on what Vic had told me. "Duke," who stands six-feet-six inches tall in his (now banned) Tony Llama anteater boots, just loves his barbecued meat and frequent chili cookouts.

But, my oh my, did he ever pay for such indulgences with every type of conceivable gut ache imaginable. Now "Duke" isn't one for health food as such. "I don't like that sissy stuff only nerds and whimps eat!" he brags loudly whenever we get on the subject of nutrition. "I like real he-man food—the kind that sticks to your ribs and fills your belly!"

At first he was a bit reluctant, I'll have to admit, about trying something with which he was totally unfamiliar. But I had him invest the time, energy, and funds into growing his own fennel and then getting himself a Vita-Mix juicer to make it in. Only after his wife started doing this for him and he began drinking tiny amounts of it with every big meal he put away, did he begin to feel more comfortable inside.

I don't think I'll ever be able to change Vic's or "Duke's" eating habits. No more than President Bill Clinton is apt to become a Republican. But at least I was able to find a remedy from the first individual to help the second person. That is enough of an accomplishment right there, to make me feel somewhat satisfied.

Anxiety Attacks; Hysteria; Psychosis.   Many plant juices are intended to be drunk; but a very few are meant to be *smelled* and *slowly savored* BEFORE being swallowed. Fennel is one of these. The smell of fennel is very delicate, aromatic, and pleasant, while the taste of the herb is agreeably sweet and pleasing to the palate. Fennel juice, it may be said, combines all of these and should be held just under the nostrils and gently sniffed for a few minutes in between short sips. With each sip the tongue should slowly savour every wonderful moment before the juice is finally swallowed. This method of drinking fresh fennel juice is especially recommended for those suffering serious mental attacks of fear or suspicion. There is something unique in the licorice-like flavor and taste of this remarkable herb that calms the mind and soothes the conscience. The two principal constituents are anethole (50-60%) and fenchone (18-22%). Anethole is also the chief constituent in anise. When the human senses of smell and taste come into contact with these two principals, a chemical reaction takes place in the limbic portion of the brain— that area known as the "pleasure center" of the mind. The authors of *The Pleasure Connection*, both of them Registered Nurses and husband-and-wife, explain how the production of endorphins is triggered within the body by foods such as fennel juice. Once these "feel-good" peptides are released into the blood stream, they work in a way similar to opium in that they create a mood of euphoria and essentially dampen feelings of suspicion and fear. This is how fennel juice is able to achieve this remarkable action.

(Deva Beck, R.N. and James Beck, R.N. *The Pleasure Connection: How Endorphins Affect Our Health and Happiness* (San Marcos, CA: Synthesis Press, 1987.)

Gallstones.   A woman named Mrs. Stephens in 18th century England developed a cure for gallstones with fresh fennel juice as one of her key ingredients. She had such astonishing success with it, that a special Act of Parliament was passed in 1739, so that the secret of the preparations used might be made known to the public. She received a lifetime reward of 5,000 pounds, a goodly sum of money in that time. Her recipe was eventually published in the *London Gazette*, June 19, 1739.

METHOD OF PREPARATION

Pick yourself six fennel stems, leaves, and flowers. Separate the leaves and flowers from the stems, and discard the latter. Wash the leaves and flowers in a coarse wire sieve before juicing. If using a Vita-Mix, add a little celery or carrot juice to help the other juice taste better. Remember—a *little* bit goes a *long* way!

GARLIC-ONION JUICE

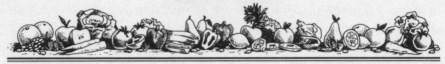

"Treatment for Burns, Fungus, and Arteriosclerosis/Atherosclerosis"

DESCRIPTION

Garlic (*Allium sativum*) is a hardy perennial plant. It is the most potent and pungent member of the onion family. The plant grows to a height of almost a foot and produces delicate white flowers. The plant produces segmented bulbs of very strong onion-like flavor. Each bulb, called a head or a knob, contains eight to twelve sections, called cloves. These cloves are covered and held closely together by a parchmentlike covering. The garlic plant doesn't produce seeds but is propagated by planting the cloves. There are three basic types of garlic: Creole, Italian (Mexican), and Tahitian.

Most of our garlic is supplied from California, and since these supplies are supplemented by imports from the Southern Hemisphere, garlic is in ample supply year-round. Nearly all the California garlic is of the Creole variety, which features fair-sized heads, white skins, fairly large cloves, and a fairly mild flavor. The Italian (Mexican) garlic has a purplish skin and is smaller in size than the California (Creole) variety. It has smaller cloves but a sharper flavor. The Tahitian variety has an insignificant share of the total market. This variety produces extra-large heads and is often called elephant garlic.

These white heads are at least twice as large as those found in the other two types. Tahitian garlic has a milder flavor and is usually sold by specialty shops or mail-order houses at three or four times the price of the smaller garlic.

Shop for garlic as you would for onions. Ignore the white or purplish color of the parchmentlike skin; both types are of equal quality. Select firm, dry, sprout-free heads. Garlic shows age by getting soft or wet and by shooting green sprouts. Unlike the onion, which has to be used quite soon after it has been cut, you can remove as little as a single clove of garlic without decreasing the lasting power of the remaining cloves.

The onion (*Allium cepa*) is a hardy biennial of the lily family, grown for its immature stems, which are sold as green or bunch onions, and its ripe, firm bulbs. These bulbs come in various shapes and colors and with different degrees of pungency. The onion contains much sugar and varying amounts of mustard oil. The bulb is closely packed leaf-bases and the long, slender, tubular blades are fleshy and dark green. The flower stalk is tubular and fleshy and produces a globular head of very small greenish-white flowers, or the seed stalk may have, in place of the flowers, clusters of small onions which may be used as seed for new plants.

The common garden onion is a native of Persia. Its principal varieties are: the whites, the yellows, and the red to brown varieties. Most of the white onions are of varieties that produce a very small bulb. They are primarily boiled and used in recipes that call for creamed onions. There are also some very large white onions that are called white Spanish onions and Bermuda onions. The red-skinned, red-fleshed onions are known as Creole onions and are used primarily in salads.

The mildness or the sharpness of an onion can't be determined by its color or outward appearance, but rather by the variety and the area in which it was produced. For instance, the seed used to grow large Spanish-type onions in Idaho produces a sharper onion when produced in New York. This is also true of the imported red Italian onions, which are sweeter than those grown in Michigan or New York.

There are also several types of onions known for their sweetness and mildness. Leading contenders for this category would include the Vidalia onions grown in Georgia, the Maui onions grown in

Hawaii, and the Walla Walla onions grown in Washington State. All three are fine products of comparable quality and flavor, but they usually sell at premium prices. However, the less-heralded onions grown in Texas, California, and the Pacific Northwest are almost, if not just as, sweet and mild as those and a lot less expensive.

Look for very firm, dry, well-shaped onions that are almost free from odor and completely free from sprouting. Softness at the neck (the top) of the onion is a dead giveaway as to impending or actual decay. Onions should always be stored in a cool, dry area.

Another member of the allium family, the shallot (*Allium ascalonicum*), at first glance looks like a very small, old yellow onion but it is actually one of the most elegant members of the onion clan. The dull, copper-colored, parchment-skinned exterior hides a very distinctive flavor that is somewhere between that of garlic and onion. The shallot is highly prized by French chefs.

Some years ago the Wakunaga Pharmaceutical Company of Hiroshima, Japan, began experimenting with various types of garlic, until it had selected one kind that suited its manufacturing needs. Ever since then this garlic has been grown in abundance in the northern part of Japan in ground that has been previously enriched with seaweed, fish protein, and mineral powders. The result is an incredibly nutritious garlic, which after being harvested and temporarily dried, is then put into huge oil refinery-like tanks and allowed to "age" for many months. This special "aging" process dramatically increases the vitamin, enzyme, and trace element contents of the garlic, while at the same time considerably reducing its objectionable odor.

This Japanese aged garlic extract is sold in the United States under the brand name of Kyolic. There is a liquid version sold in a two fluid ounce bottle in most health food stores nationwide, and has been enriched with vitamins B_1 and B_{12}. I recommend using this instead of juicing raw garlic cloves. There are several reasons for this. First, a small but significant number of individuals are allergic to the oils and smell of raw garlic, and experience bad reactions to them. Secondly, raw garlic is very hypoglycemic and will produce untoward effects in people suffering from low blood sugar. Thirdly, due to the tiny size of the cloves themselves, juicing raw garlic can prove to be a real challenge. All of these problems are resolved, however, when you substitute raw garlic juice with the liquid Kyolic aged garlic extract.

When juicing onions, I recommend the Vidalia or Walla Walla for their sweetness, a little shallot for extra flavor and some green bunch onions. The liquid Kyolic garlic extract can then be included with the juice of the others. Because onion and garlic juices in combination with each other can be somewhat overpowering even for the bravest souls, I strongly advise juicing some fresh bunch parsley in with them. This way the flavor becomes more tolerable without compromising the wonderful medicinal properties of the alliums being used.

Onions

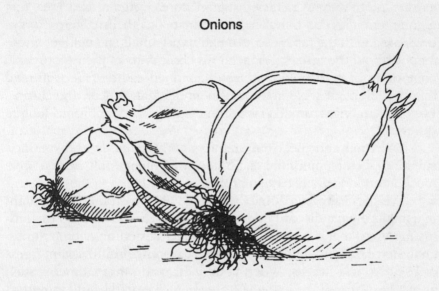

NUTRITIONAL DATA

The chemistry of garlic, onion, and shallot is incredibly complex, more so for the first than the latter two. In looking for the nutrients that are present in them, our attention should not be focused so much on their vitamin content as on their incredibly rich trace element contents. Garlic and onion contain three very important minerals, namely sulphur, potassium, and germanium in that order. The amount of potassium in one clove of garlic or one tablespoon of minced onion will average about 16 milligrams, while the germanium content will range anywhere from one to four parts per billion (ppb), according to the *Chemical & Pharmaceutical Bulletin* (28:2691, 1980).

The first serious epidemiologic study relating potassium to blood pressure was published in 1959, based on medical research conducted in two villages in northern Japan. Since then, a great deal more information has appeared in the medical literature showing a definite connection between high potassium intake and a reduction in elevated blood pressure levels. Important data presented at the First World Garlic Congress held several years ago in Washington, D.C. has confirmed the therapeutic role of garlic in treating hypertension. Undoubtedly the potassium in it has accounted for some of this effect.

In the last few years, germanium has captured tabloid headlines as one of the "new miracle vitamin cures." Again, the idea that germanium may be beneficial to human health in different ways originated with the Japanese. A metallurgist and coal engineer wrote a book about the research done at his clinic with a synthetic organic compound of germanium. More research since then has confirmed this trace element's role in the treatment of AIDS, cancer, and chronic Epstein-Barr virus or EBV syndrome (which is a chronic fatigue disorder).

The final and most important mineral in garlic and onion is sulphur. Doctors, nutritionists, and health writers don't seem to give much attention to this particular trace element.

I've spent almost a decade studying this tremendously important mineral and have discovered in all of the research surveyed (including my own) that it is *the key* to preventing hardening of the arteries, cholesterol buildup in the heart, and to stopping drug-resistant forms of bacteria and fungus. When combined with other elements such as potassium and germanium in spices like garlic and onion, a powerful trio of *chelating* agents are formed which keep the heart and liver free of fatty deposits, the immune defenses alert and active, and the condition of the skin healthy and young.

THERAPEUTIC BENEFITS

In the *Salt Lake Tribune* (Thursday, January 23, 1986, p. A-11) some years ago appeared this item in Ann Landers' syndicated newspaper column from an Oklahoma couple:

> "Our 11-month-old son was sitting on my lap at the dinner table while we were having dessert and coffee. All of a sudden little Albert jarred my hand and the hot coffee went right down the front of his chest.

"My husband grabbed Albert and stripped off his shirt. I put on some cold towels and that quieted him. A friend who was having dinner with us ran and chopped up some onions and applied them to the boy's burns. We took turns walking the floor with him. A couple of hours later he was perfectly quiet, as if nothing had happened. I rocked him to sleep and he slept through the night..." Ann Landers mocking reply was something to this effect:

"You and your husband should have taken the child to an emergency room of a hospital with the cold towels (and ice) on his chest. (What's with the chopped onions? Never heard of such a thing.)"

I wrote a letter to Ann Landers the same day her column appeared with this item in it. I called her attention to a fascinating scientific report in an old medical journal. I suggested that one of her staff go to the University of Illinois's medical library and check out *Bulletin of the History of Medicine* (15:143-48, February 1944), which contains an article entitled, "Ambroise Paré's Onion Treatment of Burns" by Henry E. Sigerist. I went on to then explain how a French surgeon named Paré (1510–1590) discovered one of the best medicines for treating all manner of burns.

"Paré was a keen observer," wrote Sigerist. "As a surgeon who had not studied in a university, he did not share the academic bias of many contemporary physicians and relied on his own observations rather than on reasoning along traditional lines. Like Paracelsus he was always on the alert, eager to learn from any, even the humblest source." Sigerist then proceeds to tell how Paré came by the onion discovery. It was at Piedmont, France around 1537. As a young surgeon of 27 years of age, he was attached to the army of the Marshal de Montejan in the third war between Francis I and Charles V. One of Montejan's kitchen boys accidentally fell into a cauldron of boiling hot oil and was severely burned.

I will now let Paré himself speak in regard to what happened next. (This is quoted in Sigerist's article.)

"I being called to dress him, went to the next Apothecaries to fetch refrigerating medicines commonly used in this case. Now there was present by chance a certain old country woman, who hearing that I desired medicines for a burn, persuaded me at the first dressing, that I should lay on rags soaked in raw onion juice mixed with a little salt, saying that I would hinder the breaking out of blister or pustules, as she had found by certain and frequent experience. Wherefore I

thought good to try the force of her medicine upon this greasy scullion.
I the next day found those places of his body whereto the onions lay,
to be free from blisters, but the other parts which they had not touched,
to be all blistered."

Although Ann Landers did not print my response, she nevertheless acknowledged my letter with a form letter of appreciation.
Since reading this some years ago in the Eccles Health Sciences
Library at the University of Utah Medical Center, I've had numerous
occasions to recommend and personally use this onion juice-salt
therapy for sunburns and first-, second-, and third-degree burns with
much success! I can testify that it works just as well as anything a
hospital might use for such emergency situations.

The use of fresh garlic juice for even the worst type of fungal
infection is best illustrated with two separately published case studies
from India: "Sporotrichosis treated with garlic juice," which appeared
in the *Indian Journal of Dermatology* (28:42–45, January 1983); and
"Lymphatic fungal infection cured with garlic juice" (*Folk Medicine
Journal* 1:118–119, Spring 1993). In both instances, cases of inter-
nal/external fungus in soldiers serving in the Indian Army were
successfully treated with raw garlic juice, when more conventional
antibiotic drug therapies failed. In both studies, areas of the infected
skin treated with garlic juice dressings showed remarkable and quick
improvements, while other areas treated with synthetic medications
showed little, if any, improvements.

A study conducted in Japan by scientists from the Wakunaga
Pharmaceutical Co. (makers of Kyolic garlic) and published in the
March, 1987 issue of *Applied and Environmental Microbiology*
(53:615–17) explained how a particular sulphur compound in garlic,
called ajoene, dramatically inhibited fungal growth. This evidence
clearly demonstrates that nothing is better for *any* kind of fungal
infection than garlic juice.

Besides the numerous published reports from leading scientists
in different countries showing that garlic and onion can significantly
lower serum cholesterol and triglyceride levels, there is additional
proof, albeit anecdotal, in support of this fact. Henry Wascombe is a
court magistrate in England. David Roser, author of *Garlic For Health*
and himself a resident of Bury St. Edwards, Suffolk, England, made
me familiar with Mr. Wascombe's case awhile back at the World Garlic
Congress in Washington, D.C.

Mr. Wascombe, it seems, developed a severe case of arterioscle-rosis, which involved a buildup of calcium deposits on the inside of the artery walls of his heart. This produced a thickening and hardening of the arteries. At some point, his condition advanced to a more severe type of hardening (atherosclerosis) when fatty deposits began accumulating in these same walls and contributed to a degeneration of the arteries themselves.

When Magistrate Wascombe started experiencing hypertension, temporary muscle paralysis, chest pressure, and pains that radiated from his chest to his left arm and shoulder, he consulted with several specialists to see what the problem was. Numerous x-rays were taken and tests made, with the final prognosis given as previously stated. Some doctors felt that even surgery might prove to be a risky venture, considering what bad shape his heart was in.

Feeling especially glum, the judge decided he had nothing to lose by conferring with a medical herbalist. (In Great Britain medical herbalists are protected under a special charter granted to them several centuries ago, which allows them to diagnose and prescribe just as regular doctors can. They receive extensive training in herbal lore and general medicine before receiving their licenses to practice.) The individual to whom Magistrate Wascombe presented himself prescribed five tablespoons of a garlic-and-onion mix (equal parts of each) every day. In addition, his lady herbalist put him on tinctures of mistletoe, belladonna, and Crataegus (hawthorn).

Within six months, David related, the judge's symptoms had just about all disappeared. He had more energy and vitality, was able to engage in some strenuous physical activity without pain, could breathe freely, and "felt like a new man again!"

Encephalitis.   This condition usually involves infection by herpes simplex virus, meningitis virus, or other viruses of like severity. Transmission can be through human or animal contact or a bite from a mosquito or tick carrying any of these viruses. The condition is marked by severe inflammation of the brain. The role of heavy garlic-onion juice therapy here is that both agents contain very potent sulphur compounds, which work in the brainstem gray matter and the cerebral cortex and anterior horn cells of the spinal cord where most of the infection is likely to be.

Meningitis. Meningitis is a dread complication of a particularly nasty infection induced by the fungus *Coccidioides immitis*, which is common in the arid West and Southwest. It seems to favor Caucasians more than other ethnic groups. Bone and joint lesions, skin ulcers, and organ involvement are apparent. Another type of fungus, *Cryptococcus neoformans*, which has worldwide distribution, causes another type of meningitis. It is most common in individuals undergoing chemotherapy and radiation for existing cancers and in those suffering from Hodgkin's disease. This organism has been isolated from the upper respiratory tracts of many healthy people in Southeast Asia. But the intriguing reason as to why they remain free of this disease is because they *regularly chew and use raw garlic.* In one of my recently published books, *From Pharoahs to Pharmacists: The Healing Benefits of Garlic* (New Canaan, CT: Keats Publishing, Inc., 1994; p. 107) I mention a report from the *Chinese Medical Journal* (93: 123, Feb. 1980) in which a garlic juice extract was given orally for several weeks to 21 patients suffering from *Cryptococcal meningitis.* In 11 of the patients there was noticeable improvement; and of these 6 were totally cured!

Worms. Intestinal parasites thrive in the gut and colon of many human beings. Raw garlic and onion therapy has been extremely beneficial in removing these worms. The strong sulphur compounds in both culinary herbs overwhelm the parasites, often knocking them into a stupor via their vapors, or else totally immobilizing them by "poisoning" the circulating blood plasma around them from which they derive their nourishment. While in such temporary paralysis, they are no longer able to cling to intestinal tissue walls, thereby enabling the body to throw them off in normal bowel movements.

METHOD OF PREPARATION

As mentioned before, I suggest that the liquid extract of Kyolic aged garlic be substituted in lieu of raw garlic juice, because of the adverse reactions which a small but statistically significant number of people have to it. To every one-fourth cup onion juice, I recommend adding a level teaspoon of the Kyolic liquid garlic.

After peeling an onion, cut it in half with a French knife, then quarter it. If using something like a Vita-Mix to juice with, I'd cut these quarters into small bits for easier juicing purposes. Some green onions, washed and cleaned, should also be juiced with them. As previously stated, a half bunch of parsley or some fresh watercress or spinach leaves should be juiced and then mixed with the garlic-onion to make it more palatable.

Another way to juice garlic cloves is to wrap them in some kale leaves and then push them through the hopper of your juice machine with a carrot. In fact, one garlic clove, one small piece of a sweet Vidalia onion, two each broccoli flowerets, kale leaves, carrots, and tomatoes, and pinches of cayenne pepper and granulated kelp make one dynamic vegetable cocktail. These can all be juiced together and then thoroughly blended.

When attempting to use garlic-onion juice on serious burns, put on some new plastic gloves. Then take strips of gauze and soak them in a juice solution of both. Lift each strip out with one hand and using two fingers of the other, lightly run down either side of the gauze to get out excess liquid. Then loosely apply to the burn area and secure in place.

When used externally to get rid of fungal infection, tape together several cotton Q-tips and soak one end in some garlic-onion juice. Then work on, into, or beneath the area of skin or nail thus afflicted. If using it internally for fungal problems, such as in the mouth, either gargle or else brush the gums and tongue with some of the juice. It can also be used as a douche to combat vaginitis, or gently warmed in a metal spoon over a flame and a few drops put into the ears to stop infection and earache.

GRAPE-RAISIN JUICES

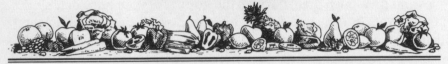

"Putting Herpes into Hibernation"

DESCRIPTION

No other fruit that I know of has excited such interest in me over the years as grapes (*Vitis* species). The ancients had quite a bit to say about this particular fruit in many of their writings, some of which have survived in different forms. The single most fascinating thing they all seem to agree on is that *the grape was the 'forbidden fruit' eaten by Adam and Eve in the Garden of Eden.*

    Some of the many different sources I have drawn on for this likely fact are as follows:

R. H. Charles. *The Apocrypha and Pseudepigrapha of the Old Testament* (Oxford: University Press, 1976), II:535-36 (III Baruch 4:8-15).

Rabbi Dr. H. Freedman and Maurice Simon. *Midrash Rabbah* (London: The Soncino Press, 1961), I:151 (Genesis 14:5).

The Babylonian Talmud: Sanhedrin II (London: The Soncino Press, 1935), II:478 (70a-70b).

Isidore Singer (Ed.). *The Jewish Encyclopedia* (New York: Funk & Wagnalls Co., 1903), 6:81.

The Nag Hammadi Library in English (San Francisco: Harper & Row, 1977), pp. 110-111; 127; 143-144; 154; 168

The question then arises, "Why was it *specifically* the grape that Adam and Eve consumed? Why couldn't it have been some other type of fruit instead?" This leads us back again to ancient traditions as to the likely backgrounds of earth's first couple. Eliza R. Snow, a very gifted poetess, penned these lines regarding both of them in her epic poem, "The Ultimatum of Human Life." She was, of course, merely borrowing knowledge already understood by the ancients when she wrote:

> Adam, your God, like you on earth, has been Subject to sorrow in a world of sin: Through long gradation he arose to be Cloth'd with the Godhead's might and majesty... By his obedience he obtain'd the place *Of God and Father of this human race!*

> Obedience will the same bright garland weave, As it has done for your great Mother, Eve, ... What did she care, when in her lowest state, Whether by fools, consider'd small, or great? 'Twas all the same with her—she prov'd her worth—*She's now the Goddess and the Queen of Earth!*

> [Eliza R. Snow. *Poems. Religious, Historical, andPolitical* (Salt Lake City: 1877), pp. 8-9.]

Assuming then that such traditions are correct, it would imply that when Adam and Eve came from Heaven to this world, they came as perfect, holy, and resurrected beings, constituting flesh, bone, and spirit but *lacking* blood because they were still immortals. *The Nag Hammadi Library in English* (pp. 168-169) sheds some light on *why* the grape was chosen as the "forbidden fruit." "Therefore, those who drink it [grape juice] acquire for themselves the desire for intercourse," reads the translated text. The ancients held to the notion that since there was no sexuality in Heaven, a "forbidden fruit" of some kind (like the grape) had to be created to stimulate sexual desires in each other, which, in turn, produced not only blood in this heavenly couple, but also allowed them to have *mortal* children as well, *outside* the sacred confines of the Garden of Eden. Once they had "lived" long enough to see this satisfactorily accomplished, they re-entered the Garden in an old and decrepit state. There, so Nag Hammadi text goes, they partook of "clusters of *white* grapes" from "the tree of life" with color like that of the sun. After consuming adequate quantities of these particular grapes for an unspecified period of time, their bodies became young and eternal again, which enabled them to ascend back into Heaven and reclaim their thrones of power and glory. At least such is the stuff of which intriguing and thrilling legends about the grape have been made in ancient times and periodically readapted in ages since.

Grapes grow on gnarled, woody, climbing vines with peeling bark. Grape leaves are palmately lobed, usually medium-green to blue-green, lush, and dramatic, turning yellow in the fall.

The plants can be trained to climb on or to cling to many different structures. Grape arbors are something special to sit under and smell the ripening grapes, to just reach up and pluck a few ripe ones, or merely to lean back and enjoy a glass of homemade wine—now that's fine living, indeed!

Four major classes of grapes are grown in the United States: the American grape, the European grape, the muscadine, and the hybrids of the three named. American grapes are native to the Northeast and are grown in bunches, have skins that slip off easily, and are generally eaten fresh or made into jelly, juice, and occasionally wine. European grapes have tight skins and a typically winey flavor. They separate into three main categories: those used for wine, the dessert grapes, and the *raisin* grapes. Muscadine grapes, best characterized by the 'scuppernong,' are native to the Southeast. They grow in loose clusters, have a slightly musky flavor, and are eaten fresh or made into jelly and occasionally into a fruity wine. Many hybrids have been developed which combine many of the characteristics of the American, European, and muscadine grapes.

The raisin is our most important dried fruit and is produced by drying grapes in sunlight. Ninety-nine percent of our raisins are seedless, all of which are made from Thompson seedless grapes. Golden-colored seedless raisins are nothing more than regular raisins that have been bleached with sulphur dioxide. Cluster raisins that have seeds and are attached to the stems are made from muscatel grapes. They used to be fairly popular in our grandparents' time, but have all but disappeared from the marketplace. Those tiny Zante currants that are frequently used by bakers for muffins aren't really currants at all. They are tiny raisins made from the petite seedless black Corinth grapes.

When shopping for table grapes it is imperative to remember that the fruit doesn't ripen any further or improve in flavor after it has been severed from the vine. What you see, or better yet what you taste, if you are permitted to sample the grapes at the time of purchase, is what you get. The quicker you use them the better; as they age they lose crispness and flavor.

Look for firm, plump, colorful, dry berries that are firmly attached to pliable green stems. A professional buyer checks out the freshness of the grapes by examining the amount of bloom on the berry. Bloom is the name given to the waxy, powderlike coating applied by nature to protect the fruit from the direct rays of the sun. This coating is more obvious on the darker-colored grapes, but it is also present, though not as easily detected, on the light-colored varieties. The heavier the bloom, the fresher the grape. As the grape starts to age and break down (after one to two weeks), the bloom disappears. Color is very important, especially in the green varieties. The greener the grape, the lower the sugar content. The yellower the grape, the higher the sugar content. Red varieties are at their best when the berries are predominantly of high color. The darker the blue grapes, the better the quality.

Table grapes may make lovely centerpiece table attractions but will soon start to break down at room temperature. They must be kept in the refrigerator immediately after purchase until used up. The crispness and the flavor of the grapes are enhanced when they are fully chilled.

NUTRITIONAL DATA

One cup of grape juice contains: 28 mg. calcium, 30 mg. phosphorus, 0.8 mg. iron, 5 mg. sodium, 293 mg. potassium, and small amounts of vitamins A, B-complex, C, and P. One cup of unpacked raisins yields: 90 mg. calcium, 146 mg. phosphorus, 5.1 mg. iron, 39 mg. sodium, 1,106 mg. potassium, 30 I.U. vitamin A, and traces of B-complex and C.

THERAPEUTIC BENEFITS

Five years ago in Costa Mesa, California I spoke to a "Herpes Awareness Group," as they called themselves. They consisted of mostly middle-class, upwardly mobile yuppies in their late twenties and thirties, who shared one thing in common, namely the herpes simplex virus. I was invited there to present new information about controlling this nasty and complex microbe with natural substances.

I remember citing a study which was published in the December, 1976 issue of *Applied and Environmental Microbiology* (32:757-63) in which two Canadian microbiologists reported that Concord and seedless grape juices and red and white wines were able to inhibit cholera, herpes simplex, and influenza viruses, among others. I then spoke of my own research with raisin juice, that is the juice of cooked raisins, and how it helped in the management of some cases of herpes simple I virus.

Not long after this, a woman by the name of Mallory K. wrote to me, explaining how my remarks prompted her to try grape juice for her own herpes. "I quickly discovered that commercially bottled grape juice didn't do much for me," she said. "I assumed it was due to the juice being heated before it was bottled. So I started to make fresh grape juice myself. I began with the seedless grapes first, because they seemed a lot easier to work with. By experimenting around a little I found out that the dark grapes worked the best. I juiced them with their seeds and then strained the liquid afterwards through some layers of fine muslin. It took only one cup of the *fresh dark* grape juice each day to bring my herpes condition under control." She mentioned that she had shared this find with some of her friends similarly afflicted, and they, too, reported it working well for them.

Years ago there was a book written by Johanna Brandt entitled *The Grape Cure*, in which the marvelous properties of grapes and grape juice were highly touted for curing *any* kind of cancer. The book became somewhat of a best-seller in its time and tens of thousands of people suffering from cancer went on this particular juice therapy.

How successful this was, may be better judged from the following true episode. A couple of years ago I purchased a nice leather-bound set of rare books from a prolific fundamentalist Mormon writer named Ogden Kraut, who was retired from his previous occupation as a photographer at the Tooele Ordinance Depot west of Salt Lake City. (This is only one of several facilities in the country where the U.S. Army conducts top-secret germ warfare tests on animals in very confined environments. Mr. Kraut's job was to photograph these animals in their varying stages of decrepitude, while wearing an oversized "space suit" to protect himself from coming into contact with these extremely deadly viruses.)

At the time I made this business transaction with him, he informed me he was just recovering from the effects of a very malignant cancer which had been discovered in his abdomen. The doctors wanted to do surgery and give him massive doses of chemotherapy and radiation, but, in so many words, he plainly told them to "go to hell" and decided to treat the problem himself. Kraut went on a very lengthy fast of some months, subsisting mostly on grape juice and a fruit-and-vegetable diet.

He stated that his tumor began going into remission within weeks of his radical diet change. He stayed on this juice therapy until later x-rays showed that the cancer was totally gone. He, of course, lost considerable weight, but claimed, "I felt great and had more energy than I've had in years. I felt like a young kid all over again. My mind was sharp, my energy levels incredible and I slept like a log!" Whether or not grape juice will do the same thing for someone else's cancer remains to be seen. But certainly it occupies an important position in a comprehensive nutritional program designed to combat cancer.

Fatigue.   If a person is lacking adequate energy and isn't troubled with blood sugar problems, then grapes and raisins might be just the ticket. Both are high in natural sugar content; raisins have an additional bonus of iron, which is an important blood nutrient for women. Grape-raisin juice works primarily in the liver where most of the body's energy production takes place.

Heart Attack.   On the 25-year award-winning television news program "60 Minutes" for Sunday, November 11, 1991, veteran correspondent Morley Safer reported on "The French Paradox." He introduced his topic by pointing out that several things are known to contribute to heart attacks, poor diet being one of them. "So why is [it]," he asked, "that the French, who eat 30% more fat than we do, suffer fewer heart attacks, even though they smoke more and exercise less [than we do]?" He noted that the gastronomy of the French culture is enough to "send the American Heart Association into cardiac arrest—butter, goose fat, lard, double cream are the staples of a decent day's cooking." The French health "secret" against heart attacks, as it turns out, is red wine and grape juice. The French drink a lot of both with their typically artery clogging meals. Red wine and Concord grape juice both have a definite flushing action on artery walls, to help remove blood platelets that cling to rough, fatty plaque, which can cause clogging and blockage that produces a sudden heart attack.

Viral Infections.   Two Canadian microbiologists published an important piece of research in the scientific journal *Applied and Environmental Microbiology* (32:757-63, Dec. 1976). Appropriately entitled, "Virus inactivation by grapes and wines," their report presented documented evidence to show that the high concentration of tannins in these fruits were potent killers of disease-causing viruses in test tubes. The two researchers bought grapes, grape juice, and raisins from local grocery stores, and red, rose, and white wines in Ottawa, Quebec Province. They then added viruses to the grape extract made from pulp and skins, to the grape juice and infusions of raisins, and to the wines. All inactivated the viruses. Grape juice was especially potent against poliovirus and herpes simplex virus, causes of polio and herpes infections respectively.

METHOD OF PREPARATION

Because nearly all commercial grapes sold in supermarkets today are heavily sprayed with pesticides, I'm somewhat ambivalent about recommending them for juicing purposes. Your best bet, if possible, is to locate sources of *organically* grown grapes. Washing them off simply won't do, as most of these chemicals penetrate directly *into* the grape skin. Unlike apples, oranges, or bananas, which you can either peel or wash with soap and water, grapes that have been sprayed are a little different.

If there is no other choice available but to use commercially grown grapes, then be sure to juice just enough for half a cup of juice each day and *no more than this.* Also taking some dandelion root (3) and yucca (2) capsules *with* the grape juice should help to minimize the risk of the pesticides in it.

Wash the grapes to be used and remove their stems. Then run them through your juicer on a medium speed setting. If using red grapes, strain the juice through a fine-wired strainer to remove the seeds that may have come through intact. If using seedless grapes, however, this isn't necessary to do.

A nice grape-melon-raisin slush can be made that will not only prove tasty but will also help control milder forms of the herpes virus. Put one cup of packed raisins into three-fourth quart of water. Bring to a slow boil, then reduce the heat to a lower setting and simmer, covered, for one hour. Then strain the juice and pour into an ice cube tray and set in the freezer until hard.

Next take one and one-half pounds seedless green grapes (four cups) and wash them in a large colander and remove their stems. Place the grapes in a Vita-Mix or similar blender and puree. Pour this puree into a coarse wire strainer placed over a mixing bowl and press with the back of a wooden ladle or spoon to extract as much juice as possible. There should be about two cups of juice. Discard the pulp.

Remove the seeds from the melon and scoop the flesh into the Vita-Mix or blender. Process until liquefied; you should have about two cups of juice. Add the melon juice to the grape juice, cover the bowl and refrigerate the mixture for three hours to allow both flavors to nicely meld together.

Take out the tray from the freezer and place the raisin juice ice cubes in a heavy-duty plastic bag, and pound them with a wooden mallet until they are sufficiently broken into almond-size pieces. Then place these pieces in the juicer or blender and process for 15 to 30 seconds, or until finely crushed.

Then scoop one-half cup of this crushed raisin juice ice into a regular drinking glass and pour one cup of the melon-grape juice into the glass. You have an unusual drink with a unique flavor that will taste good and be good for you.

HORSERADISH JUICE

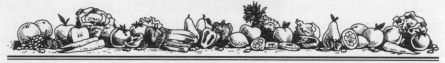

"Very Potent Remedy for Hypothermia"

DESCRIPTION

"Horses' radish" (*Armoracia rusticana*) is what an old ornery cook named Roy Elliott, with whom I worked many years ago at Elliott's Cafe in Provo, Utah, used to call this herb. This unattractive and sometimes weedy plant is a member of the mustard family. It is prized for its large fleshy roots, which are ground and used as a dressing for meats. It has a very strong, sharp, pungent flavor, and it is usually diluted with vinegar.

The plant makes a rosette of long leaves, which are two to three inches wide and over a foot long. It has a flower-stalk two to three feet tall, with small white flowers. Native to the Mediterranean regions, it has become a weed in many sections of the globe. It's not a particularly good plant for the casual gardener, as it will spread out and dominate garden space and is very hard to eradicate. A large amount of the commercial crop of horseradish is grown in the Mississippi Valley particularly in Missouri. Some horseradish is also grown on the Eastern Seaboard.

144

NUTRITIONAL DATA

One teaspoon of raw, freshly ground horseradish root is very high in sulphur and potassium, with medium amounts of sodium, calcium, phosphorus (in that order), and trace amounts of iron, magnesium, copper, and vitamins A, B-complex, C, and E.

THERAPEUTIC BENEFITS

Lydia Maria Child was no ordinary compiler of household hints. Newspaperwoman, magazine editor, novelist, poet, reformer, she was the foremost woman of her day, a friend of Whittier, Lowell, and Bryant. Editor and chief contributor for the first juvenile periodical in America, she was the unsung author of "Over the river and through the woods, to grandmother's house we go." No doubt the poem was a nostalgic reference to her childhood in New England, where she learned housewifery and the secrets of woodlore and herbs. An insatiable reader, and a schoolteacher at 18, she wrote her first novel at 22. It was an instant success, and began a literary career that could have flourished only in New England, where women authors weren't considered "odd" at all.

At the age of 25, in 1827, she married David Child, a charming dreamer whose irresponsible ways quickly scattered any royalties she earned. *The Frugal Housewife* (12th ed.) (Boston: Carter, Hendee and Co., 1832), one of her most popular works was written during the first year of their marriage, mostly from first-hand experience. They were to live most of their lives on rough farms, constantly in debt.

She learned of a particular remedy for treating hypothermia from older folks, who apparently suffered with it during the cold winters which New England is famous for. This unintentional decrease in body temperature is most common in newborns and infants and the elderly, particularly during operations. It is marked by lethargy, pink, swollen legs, feet, hands, and arms, skin very cold to the touch, and a below normal body temperature.

Mrs. Child was one of the first, if not the first author to talk about the use of horseradish for treating this particular health disorder. She recommended that fresh horseradish roots (two to four) be grated, put into a muslin bag with a tight draw-string on top and then sufficiently pounded with a wooden mallet in a large wooden bowl, until enough of the juice had been extracted. This would then be mixed with homemade vinegar (apple cider vinegar is a good substitute) and a little table salt and taken at the rate of $\frac{1}{4}$ teaspoonful three times a day between meals.

Chemical Toxicity.   A combination of equal parts (2 tablespoons each) of horseradish juice and hydrogen peroxide, taken internally, will detoxify the body of toxic chemicals. This is based on the work of Alexander Klibanov, a professor of applied biochemistry at the Massachusetts Institute of Technology. Back at the beginning of the 1980s, he discovered that the sulphur enzyme peroxidase in horse-radish juice, when mixed with an equal amount of hydrogen peroxide, could solidify deadly chemical poisons such as PCBS, or polychlorinated biphenyls, and form them into a long chain that could then be evacuated via the body's fecal material. (PCBs have made many headlines in the last two decades at dump sites from Love Canal near Niagara Falls, N.Y. to Imperial, Missouri.)

Mucus Congestion.   A very effective way of breaking up conges-tion in the head or chest is to soak both feet in hot water into which has been dissolved some Epsom salts, while at the same time taking internally 3-5 tablespoons of horseradish juice flavored with a little pure maple syrup, if necessary. The very potent sulphur vapors will strip phlegm from mucosal tissue walls and promote a rapid dis-charge of it from the body through orifices like the nose, mouth, urinary tract, and colon.

METHOD OF PREPARATION

For obtaining horseradish root juice, it is best to use a machine with a rotating cutter on the shaft. If one isn't readily available, you can use a Vita-Mix or food blender, but only after *first* grating the root. The pulp can then be mixed with a little lemon or lime juice and a few drops of fresh chili pepper juice.

This sauce should be kept refrigerated in a closed bottle or jar, so that its potency does *not* increase dramatically if left to warm up at room temperature. Only a one-eighth to one-fourth teaspoonful should be taken every four hours on an empty stomach, but only after each spoonful has been adequately moistened with more lemon or lime juice. A copious discharge of tears from the eyes and mucus from the sinus cavities may become evident. Remember to use only *very little* at a time.

KALE-COLLARD JUICES

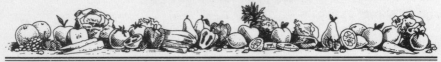

"Strengthens the Bones in Older People"

DESCRIPTION

Kale (*Brassica oleracea* var. *acephala*), a member of the cabbage family, is grown for its leaves and fleshy midribs. Kale and the Georgia collard (same Latin binomial) are probably very closely related to the wild cabbage, having been in cultivation for many centuries. It is an annual in culture, but produces its seedstalk the second year. The leaves are longer than broad, very curly, and the margins are very much cut and ruffled.

There are two types of kale: the Scotch, which has a grayish-green colored foliage, and the Siberian, which has a bluish-green color. Both tall and dwarf forms may also be had. The varieties commonly grown are the dwarf varieties, which also happen to have the greatest flavor.

Besides being a tall-growing form of kale, collard is a name also loosely applied to cabbage seedlings grown as greens and, therefore, pulled before the heads are formed. Where cabbage is successful, true collards are not very popular. They are generally grown in the South as a source of greens and as such are highly nutritious; even more so than the heading cabbage, because its leaves are entirely green.

NUTRITIONAL DATA

One cup of cooked kale yields: 206 mg. calcium, 64 mg. phosphorus, 1.8 mg. iron, 47 mg. sodium, 243 mg. potassium, 9,130 I.U. vitamin A, 1.8 mg. niacin, 102 mg. vitamin C, 23 mg. magnesium, and trace amounts of copper, manganese, and zinc. One cup of cooked collard leaves (minus the stems) contains: 357 mg. calcium, 99 mg. phosphorus, 1.5 mg. iron, 52 mg. sodium, 498 mg. potassium, 14,820 I.U. vitamin A, 2.3 mg. niacin, 144 mg. vitamin C, 31 mg. magnesium, and 1.79 mg. zinc.

THERAPEUTIC BENEFITS

On the west side of Temple Square in downtown Salt Lake City, sit two buildings opposite each other. The one on the south is the Family History Library, which is the world's largest repository of genealogical information. To the north is the LDS Church Museum.

A number of older, retired couples and single elderly adults act as volunteers in both places. Mr. and Mrs. C. Merritt, whom I met while doing research at this library, which is open to people of all faiths, work full-time and are both in their eighties. In mentioning that my next writing project would be this book, they kindly consented to sending me the following information concerning their use of kale and collard juices as a means of preventing bone fractures and breaks.

In my conversation with them (which wasn't mentioned in their subsequent letter), they related several occasions where each had slipped and fallen, either inside their apartment in the bath tub or else outside on the icy sidewalks in the winter time. Yet, "because we've been drinking these juices for years, we never experienced *any* breakage in our bones. Our doctors were, quite frankly, amazed by this, especially when they couldn't find any fractures! In fact, one doctor insisted on doing the x-rays all over again, figuring his machine wasn't working right. The only things we suffered were some bruises and having our dignities wounded."

Here is the full letter containing their incredible testimonies concerning these two marvelous vegetable juices:

11 August 1993

John Heinerman, Ph.D.
Box 11471
Salt Lake City, UT 84147

Dear Dr. Heinerman:

In response to your request that we share with you our experience with certain vegetables we are only glad to do so.

Mr. Merritt was involved with [the] production and use of dairy products since childhood. From this he suffered from undulant fever which seemed to recur whenever he used them.

In an effort to find some other source of calcium, we turned to vegetable juices. We found that kale and collards were highest on the list for garden herbs containing the bone-building minerals of calcium, phosphorus, and potassium. But when we tried to juice them sometimes we discovered that they weren't always tender or pleasant-tasting.

By experimenting around a little we soon found that they could be blended with pineapple to make a very pleasant drink. Since fresh pineapple is not always available, we substituted canned or frozen pineapple juice and sometimes added a ripe apple for good measure.

To preserve the calcium for use by the body, we quit using refined sugar products, which require so much calcium for digestion.

Presently we work full time in public service. Our average age is 83 and our health better than ever.

We appreciate your search and service in making available to us the scientific reasons for the blessing we receive by trying to apply the full "Word of Wisdom" in our lives. [The "Word of Wisdom" is a code of health revealed to the Latter-Day Saints by the Prophet Joseph Smith, Jr. It prohibits the consumption of alcohol, caffeinated beverages, and hot drinks, limits the consumption of meat only for winter and during periods of famine, denies members the use of tobacco except for medicinal purposes, and encourages the frequent use of whole grains.

Individuals who strictly adhere to this code of health enjoy long lives and are relatively disease-free.]

Sincerely,

/s/ Mr. & Mrs. C. Merritt

Many different types of health problems could be listed here, which would benefit from this kale-collards-pineapple juice mix. The reader is referred to those sections under Cabbage and Pineapple for suggested uses.

Because of the high calcium and potassium contents, the blood, heart, skin, soft tissue, muscles, kidneys, and nerves are greatly benefitted. The whopping amount of vitamin A is extremely useful in strengthening the eyes, hair, skin, soft tissue, and teeth.

Calcium Malabsorption; Osteoporosis.   The absorbable calcium levels in kale can equal or exceed the absorption levels of milk, according to research at Creighton University in Omaha, Nebraska and Purdue University in Lafayette, Indiana. For countless older women suffering from calcium deficiencies already because of malabsorption problems, this comes as good news, especially for those afflicted with brittle bones or osteoporosis. In the combined universities' study, the blood levels of calcium were actually higher in 9 of the 11 premenopausal women, when they ate cooked kale or drank the juice, than when they drank cow's milk. The kale calcium levels were pronounced as "excellent" in all 11 women just five hours after the foods were consumed. The 9 women for whom calcium absorption was higher from kale had eaten kale or drank some kale juice with a calcium content equal to that of the milk they had been consuming at an earlier phase of the study. This goes to show that vegetable calcium in items such as kale, broccoli, bok choy, and turnip, collard, and mustard greens, is more readily absorbed—and in greater quantities—than dairy calcium is.

METHOD OF PREPARATION

Mrs. Merritt said she uses an old but reliable juicer. "After running my kale and collard greens through the machine," she explained,

"I'll then run some [peeled and sectioned fresh pineapple through. I use the canned or frozen if we can't get the other. We notice that mixing one-third pineapple juice with about two-thirds of the kale-collards mix gives it a pretty delightful flavor. We usually drink a glass of this once a day with our dinner." She observed that the addition of the pineapple juice also prevents the occurrence of intestinal gas from the kale and collards.

KOHLRABI JUICE

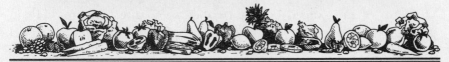

"Nothing to Sneeze at for Sinus Troubles"

DESCRIPTION

The plant kohlrabi (*Brassica cavolorapa*) is the most interesting of the cabbage family because of the structure of the stem. The leaves are similar to the turnip's, however, the stem is enlarged just above the ground to the size and shape of a turnip. The stem is really subtended by the round turnip-like structure. Kohlrabi is not grown to its full size, because when it is used before the fleshy stem gets too old, it has an excellent flavor. If grown rapidly, it is the best-flavored member of the cabbage family, with the possible exception of cauliflower. The plant seems to be of comparatively recent origin. Kohlrabi is a biennial plant which is grown as an annual in some kitchen gardens. The second year a seedstalk goes up as with other members of the cabbage clan.

Kohlrabi comes in white, green, and purple colors. The Vienna variety in any of the three colors, is generally grown. There is also an early Erfurt variety of similar quality. The white Vienna is undoubtedly the most popular.

While it is still fairly popular in Germany and central European countries, the kohlrabi has yet to achieve numerous fans in America. Yet those who sip its juice, quickly find out just how crispy the flavor is. Being so full of valuable mineral salts probably accounts for the robust alkalinity which salutes the tongue before being swallowed.

153

Select kohlrabis that look fresh and crisp and in size are no bigger than the average red beet.

NUTRITIONAL DATA

One cup of raw, diced kohlrabi contains: 57 mg. calcium, 71 mg. phosphorus, 0.1 mg. iron, 11 mg. sodium, 521 mg. potassium, 30 I.U. vitamin A, traces of B-complex vitamins, 92 mg. vitamin C, and 27 mg. magnesium.

THERAPEUTIC BENEFITS

In my professional career as a medical anthropologist, I've met a lot of ordinary people with very interesting occupations and backgrounds. One of these was a Pennsylvania woman then in her mid-thirties. She came to a holistic health conference I happened to be speaking at in the city of Philadelphia awhile back.

During the course of our conversation, this very vibrant "Jane Doe" (she didn't want her real name used) explained that her recurring sinus problems greatly interfered with her line of work. "When I can't sniff," she lamented, "I'm docked so many days' worth of pay while I'm at home recovering."

Her employer was the Butrel Chemical Senses Center, a large research institute devoted to studying all aspects of the phenomena of smell. Her particular job—and the reason, by the way, why she didn't want her real name used in this book—was that of smelling the armpits of half-clothed male volunteers or else sniffing the sweat gathered from each of them in this particular part of the body.

As goofy as her employment sounded, the research behind it was quite legitimate and made a great deal of sense. After she and other female employees had inhaled this "male essence" (as it was dubbed) for about three months, their menstrual cycles, which had ranged from less than 26 days to more than 33 days, converged around a more usual 29.5 days. Half of her fellow co-workers daubed with just alcohol on their upper lips showed no such change. Psychobiologists conducting this careful but controversial study, she told me, think they have shown that exposure to pheromones, or chemical clues, in men's armpit sweat could help adjust the female reproductive cycle to its optimal length, potentially solving some infertility problems.

I recommended that she start drinking some kohlrabi juice mixed with a little bit of carrot juice or other leafy greens. This, I pointed out in good humor, would help unclog her breathing passages enough so that she could really sense the erotic aroma in the perspiration secreted by big, beefy, and very sweaty college football linebackers. I remember her rolling her eyes around in her head at my remark, and loudly musing that "maybe I ought to be looking for something else to do."

A number of weeks passed before I heard from this lady again. Her letter expressed appreciation for the recommended remedy, stating that it had helped her immensely. "Now," she wrote, "the emphasis here [at the Butrel Chemical Senses Center] has shifted away from athletes' armpits to men's sweaty feet. I get to smell the bottoms of their feet, their sweaty socks and the insides of their shoes. A Japanese guy here hypothesizes that this type of a masculine odor might temporarily influence a female's physiology to the point that she won't get pregnant. My husband thinks it's all a bunch of nonsense, but the people I work for take these studies very seriously."

Admittedly, this "Jane Doe's" particular experience with kohlrabi juice in the line of work she's engaged in is somewhat avant-garde, to say the least. But the remedy worked well enough for her to continue making unusual sacrifices for the sake of science, and being handsomely compensated for it, too, I might add.

Bedsores; Diabetic Leg Ulcers; Gangrene; Festering Surgical Incisions and Wounds. All of these problems share one thing in common—they continually discharge foul-smelling, yellowish looking purulent matter. Kohlrabi juice made from green or purple leaves is very high in sulphur and potassium and moderately so in vitamins A and C. The sulphur amino acids and two vitamins combine to exert potent antibiotic activity against the bacteria causing such infections. In the meantime, the potassium salts are converting the highly acidic blood in which such infectious matter thrives, into a much healthier alkaline state. Routinely washing these infectious sites with kohlrabi juice externally as well as drinking enough internally, will expedite rapid healing of such deplorable problems.

METHOD OF PREPARATION

Wash and cut into small sections an average-sized kohlrabi. If using a Vita-Mix or similar blender, be sure to add a little water when liquefying so it isn't too mushy. If using another type of juicer, omit the water and juice the kohlrabi as is. Mix the juice with half cup carrot juice or some liquid chlorophyll. Most health food stores carry the powdered Kyo-Green made by Wakunaga of America, which makes a delicious and nutritious "green drink" for just about every health purpose conceivable. Including a half cup of kohlrabi juice in two-thirds glass of liquid Kyo-Green, is a good way to take this when suffering from sinus problems or other maladies.

LETTUCE JUICE

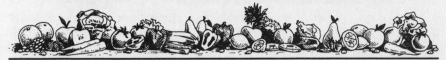

"Vegetable Narcotic for Headaches and Nervousness"

DESCRIPTION

Lettuce (*Lactuca sativa*) is probably our most popular salad plant. It is grown for its large thin leaves, which may be loose green leaves, partially folded heads, or solid heads. The plant is a native of Asia, where it was grown for centuries. It is related to the wild lettuce, with which the cultivated lettuce readily crosses. The plant is a rapidly growing annual which forms a seedstalk the same year that the heads are formed. The seedstalk may grow to three feet, with many branches terminating in several small compound flowerheads having yellow flowers.

There are four types of lettuce, three of which have been grown in America for many years. The common head lettuce (*L. sativa* var. *capitata*) is grown in greenhouses as well as in different parts of the country. The butter varieties are represented by black-seeded tennis ball, white-seeded tennis ball, and big Boston. May king belmont and bel-May are greenhouse varieties. The crisp varieties are represented by Hanson, New York, imperial, iceberg, and mignonette. There are many other varieties too numerous to mention here.

The open-head or loose-leaf type (*L. sativa* var. *crispa*) has two varieties: the butter types and the crisp kinds. The cos or romaine lettuce (*L. sativa* var. *longifolia*) forms long heads and is

157

represented by Paris white cos, green cos, dwarf, and giant white cos. Asparagus lettuce (*L. sativa* var. *angustana*) is grown for its long tender stalks.

Choosing the right kind of lettuce to buy requires a good deal more than looking for heads which are fresh, crisp and colorful. It means looking for lettuce that has been organically grown *locally* instead of purchased from the supermarket produce section. Organic lettuce from local farmers will usually be *safer* to eat than that which you buy from the store.

One of the largest and most unusual outbreaks of hepatitis A occurred in the state of Kentucky in January, 1988. The problem was considered to have reached epidemic proportions when *over* 225 people reported having contracted this deadly virus. Everywhere the same class of symptoms kept turning up in victims: unremitting nausea, lost appetite, dark urine, yellow-turning skin, and dehydration. Kentucky health authorities were so frantic that they turned to the Centers for Disease Control in Atlanta, Georgia for assistance. Though the crisis never made national news, it caused enough of a stir in Kentucky.

After much methodical medical detective work, epidemiologists were finally able to track the source of the infection. It had come from a large batch of *contaminated iceberg lettuce* which had been shipped to a number of Kentucky restaurants the week of January 16-23. Further investigation showed that the epidemic may have begun in California, which produces three-quarters of the nation's lettuce or even in Mexico. Migrant farm workers, many of whom are already infected with hepatitis A, probably relieved themselves in the lettuce fields where they had been working, and then continued to pick the crop without first washing their hands thoroughly with soap and water. (This information came from an article in the May/June, 1991 issue of *Eating Well* magazine. Since then there have been several other outbreaks of hepatitis, not on as large a scale, but still attributed to the consumption of salads in public restaurants.

Therefore, a solid piece of advice to follow is to make *very sure* that the lettuce you want to juice is *locally* grown and that those who harvest it practice reasonable hygiene. A little time and inquiry spent in this direction will yield some peace of mind and continued good health for yourself and loved ones.

Lettuce

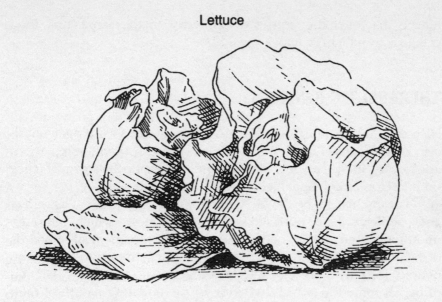

NUTRITIONAL DATA

Among several types of lettuce to choose from for juicing purposes, my own experience has taught me to prefer the romaine over the iceberg kind any day of the week. Nutritional analyses of both types bears this out. Below is a simple table showing the nutrient differences in romaine and iceberg lettuce.

LETTUCE (1 Head)	Calcium (mg.)	Phosphorus (mg.)	Iron (mg.)	Sodium (mg.)	Potassium (mg.)	Vitamin A (I.U.)	Niacin (mg.)	Vitamin C (mg.)	Magnesium (mg.)	Zinc (mg.)
Romaine	308	113	6.4	41	1,198	8,620	1.8	82	7	1
Iceberg	108	118	2.7	48	943	1,780	1.6	32	4	0.3

In every category (with the exception of sodium), romaine lettuce outranks iceberg, in some cases 3:1 as with calcium or even as much as 7:1 in vitamin A content. Romaine also has more enzyme activity, it seems, than iceberg does. I'm so disillusioned with iceberg lettuce that over the years I've ranked it in the same junk food category in which Twinkies would be.

THERAPEUTIC BENEFITS

Nicholas Culpeper (1616–1654) was a very famous astrologer-physician of the early 17th Century. After a short apprenticeship to an apothecary in St. Helen's, Bishopsgate, he set up his own practice on Red Lion Street, Spitalfields, in the year 1640.

During his life, he devoted much time to the study of astrology and medicine, and published numerous tracts, which although unorthodox and condemned by the contemporary medical standards of his time, nevertheless, enjoyed large sales among the common people. He left as his legacy to future generations a vast collection of herbal remedies, which by virtue of the undating nature of their healing properties, are as invaluable today as they were during the physician's lifetime over 340 years ago.

Culpeper was married and the father of seven children. During the Civil War which raged in England he fought on the Parliamentary side and was wounded in the chest. While his recovery was speedy enough, thanks to the many herbs he judiciously applied to his injury, he still suffered recurring headaches and nervousness.

After experimenting with different types of plants, he took some common garden lettuce leaves and pounded the juice out of them in a mortar with a stone pestle. Then in another mortar he gently crushed a number of rose petals until he obtained enough of their juice. After mixing both the lettuce and rose juices together, he rubbed some on his forehead and temples. Much to his amazement, not only did his headaches cease, but he also soon fell asleep with considerable ease.

A young lady who practices *white* witchcraft—"good witchcraft," as she calls it—in Boston, Massachusetts, read of Culpeper's remedy and decided to take it one step further. Lilith (her coven name) made separate juices from romaine leaves and rose petals, then combined them together. Next, she rubbed a little of the liquid on key acupressure points on the insides of both wrists, the palms of both hands, on both earlobes, and the bottom outsides of both ankles, and the soles of both feet. She reported that even the worst cases of stress were relieved in minutes after completing the *entire* procedure. Also when applied over the heart, liver, and stomach areas of the body, physical anxieties were removed and a calming influence soon set in.

Coughing.   During World War II codeine, an analgesic and antitussive compound, obtained from opium was in very short supply. Attention turned to a compound in lettuce called lactucarium, which has sedative and respiratory suppressant properties similar to codeine and morphine, only much weaker. For a brief period, extracts of lettuce juice were given to soldiers in need of pain relievers or cough suppressant. It seemed to work fairly well, but when codeine was again freely available, the lettuce juice extract was no longer of any interest to scientists.

Insomnia.   During the same period of time, the lactucarium from lettuce juice extract was being tested for its sedative effects on soldiers injured in battle, who were having a very difficult time sleeping on account of their pain. The lettuce juice extract worked quite well in helping them rest better, but it, too, was discontinued after World War II when other synthethic sleeping agents became more readily available and cheaper to make.

METHOD OF PREPARATION

Because the outer green leaves often contain as much as 30 percent more nutrients than the inner white leaves do, *everything* should be juiced. Don't soak the romaine in water. Many of the water-soluble vitamins can be lost this way. Instead just rinse them under running water to remove any dirt. If using a Vita-Mix, add a little cold water with the leaves. If using other popular juicers, this isn't necessary.

To either juice add some powdered kelp. The addition of a small portion (one tablespoonful to one cup juice) of this seaweed is invaluable for strengthening the adrenal glands. Rose petal juice can be made in the same way, strained and then added to the romaine-kelp juice. Diluting this juice with some distilled water before drinking it, will make the strong taste milder.

MUSTARD GREENS JUICE

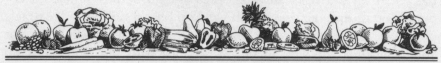

"Nutrition from the South for Women's Disorders"

DESCRIPTION

The mustards, comprising a number of plants of the genus *Brassica*, are grown throughout much of the South and a few other sections of America. They are long, broad-leaved annuals, whose leaves are used for cooking and whose seeds are used for condiments. The plants send up seedstalks, sometimes to tremendous heights, with small yellow flowers and long cylindrical pods.

There are various types and varieties of mustards. The white mustard (*Brassica alba*) whose leaves are used for potherbs, is a native of Asia. The Chinese mustard (*Brassica juncea*) is a native of Southeast Asia. In southern Russia, the seed oil has been used as a substitute for olive oil. The Japanese mustard (*Brassica japonica*) is grown to some extent in the Southern United States, for its large plume-like leaves. The black mustard (*Brassica nigra*), a native of Egypt, is grown in the southwestern part of America. In the home garden, it is grown for its leaves; commercially, for its seeds, which are the source of the mustard of commerce.

Mustard greens look like a more delicate version of kale and are a lighter green in color. These greens are a big item from Texas

162

to the Carolinas, but aren't that popular in most other states. Good mustard leaves can be dark or light green in color or even have a hint of bronze. Those which are limp and yellow are no good and should be avoided.

NUTRITIONAL DATA

One cup of mustard greens (minus their stems and leaf midribs) yields the following nutrients: 193 mg. calcium, 45 mg. phosphorus, 2.5 mg. iron, 25 mg. sodium, 308 mg. potassium, 8,120 I.U. vitamin A, 67 mg. vitamin C, 57 mg. magnesium, 2 I.U. vitamin E, 1.5 mg. zinc, and 301 mg. sulphur.

This particular herbage contains a balanced array of different nutrients essential for the health and well-being of women. Mustard greens have nearly one-quarter the recommended daily allowance (RDA) of calcium to help a woman's muscles contract better and improve her nervous system. There is almost one-quarter the RDA of iron, which helps to promote the production of more red blood cells, assists in the management of a woman's monthly menstrual cycle to keep it regular, strengthens the immune defenses to fortify her against disease, and enables her to better cope with stress. The amount of potassium present in one cup of mustard greens is enough to prevent myocardial infarction from occurring, to maintain normal blood pressure, stabilize her nervous system, and keep her heart strong. The magnesium-phosphorus balance will insure that her bones won't suffer any calcium loss soon, will keep her teeth somewhat cavity free, and increase brain function.

Much has already been discussed about the mineral sulphur under the cabbage juice section. Since a woman is more prone to rheumatoid arthritis, glandular disturbances, and hormonal imbalances than a man is, the amount of sulphur she receives by drinking a small glass of mustard greens juice every other day will help to reduce her risks of having problems. The high amount of vitamin A is especially useful for keeping her vision good, her skin soft and wrinkle-free, her hair shiny and beautiful, her teeth healthy, her bones strong, her cholesterol and blood sugar levels normal, and her immune system resistant to bacterial or viral infections.

THERAPEUTIC BENEFITS

Mavis Johnson, age 43, is a waitress in a diner on State Highway 69 just on the outskirts south of Tuscaloosa, Alabama. She heard me on a local radio talk show I did by telephone sometime ago from my home in Salt Lake City. She was one of about a dozen callers the show host and I spoke with during the hour I was on the air.

In the course of our short five minute conversation, she told us of various health problems with which she had been bothered in the past. They ranged from occasional migraines, restlessness, fatigue, and dry skin to irregular menstrual cycles, infrequent heart murmurs, periodic joint pains, and abdominal cramps. "Muh doctor told me," she said in her typical Southern drawl, "that I had a little bit of everything, but nothing serious enough to worry much about. Like I told him, 'Doc, either I am sick or I'm not sick. Don't go giving me any of this in between sickness now, you here?' So I decided to start using a remedy muh momma use to use herself whenever she felt badness like this a-creepin' all over her."

What Mavis did was to start eating cooked mustard greens—"lots of them"—put in plenty of water and drizzled with enough lemon juice for flavor. She'd save the cooking juice and drink a glass every morning before she went to work and again in the evening with supper when she returned home. "Thought you might like to know about it," she thoughtfully mused. That was when I asked what her full name, occupation, and age was. She readily gave me the first two, but then we could hear her loudly laughing in the background. "Shoot," she said, "don't you know it's bad manners to ask a lady her age?" But then she finally volunteered it.

In the meantime, I had managed to scribble down a few notes of what she had said on the back of a telephone book. I told her that I might use what she said in my next book. She laughed again and said, "Well, when you become rich and famous, you know where you can send some of that money to—right on down here to old Mavis in the diner out on South Highway 69."

Premenstrual Syndrome Pains. In some of the rural parts of Kentucky, mustard greens are boiled to the point that most of their chlorophyll juice is extracted. This is then consumed in glassfuls when cool for relieving headaches and pains generally associated with PMS.

Rheumatic Pain and Sciatica. Oldtime residents of the Appalachias have recommended to me the use of hot mustard green juice to relieve the worst rheumatic and sciatic pains imaginable. First, they make some juice out of a lot of fresh mustard greens. Those whom I visited didn't have any of the juicers mentioned in this book. Instead, they filled an old food blender or antiquated Osterizer® with one-quarter water and then added the mustard leaves, which had been finely cut with scissors. After several minutes of blending, the juice was poured into a pan and heated on the stove. Usually a teaspoonful of Ben Gay® was added to the pot and stirred in until it had completely melted. Other times a little kerosene was added to the hot juice, but only *after* it had been removed from the stove, to avoid any accidents from happening. Large square strips of clean, old bed sheets were then soaked in the mustard greens juice and applied to those parts of the body experiencing excruciating pain. An old towel or piece of flannel was then put over the pack to retain the heat longer.

METHOD OF PREPARATION

Mustard greens need to be de-stemmed and have their leaf midribs removed with a sharp knife, if you don't want the juice to be too sharp in taste. Otherwise, they can be left on and the leaves washed under running water. In a mastication juicer there is no problem using them whole, but in a centrifugal juicer such as a Vita-Mix, it's a good idea to remove stems and midribs and then cut the leaves into small pieces with a pair of scissors so they can juice more easily. It may be a good idea to add a little water with the leaves so the final liquid won't be too thick.

NECTARINE JUICE

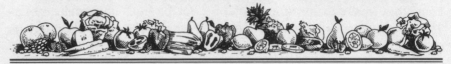

"Unbelievably Good for Your Nerves"

DESCRIPTION

The nectarine (*Prunus persica* var. *nucipersica*) originated in ancient China. It is botanically classified as a drupe and is akin to the peach, plum, apricot, and almond. While there is some difference in opinion as to whether the nectarine is a fuzzless peach, a cross between a peach and a plum, or a distinct variety, there can be no question that it is one of our finest flavored, most succulent summer fruits.

The first golden-fleshed nectarine was developed in Le Grande, California, and made its debut in 1942. More than one hundred new varieties have been developed from the original LeGrand, which was a large, not too colorful clingstone, but its claim to fame was its golden-colored flesh.

The flavor peak of the season for nectarines is June and July. The varieties that arrive then are freestone and are sweeter, juicier, and more flavorful than the clingstone varieties that come to market in August and September. People in the produce business predict that by the year 2000 the nectarine will have surpassed the peach as our number one stone fruit.

When shopping for nectarines, select those that are highly colored, velvet-skinned, unbruised and unblemished. Buy them while they are quite firm and allow them a day or two to ripen at room temperature. When they are ripe, and not before, store them in the refrigerator. The medium-sized fruit is usually the best to buy.

NUTRITIONAL DATA

One raw nectarine about two and one-half inches in diameter yields the following important nutrients: 6 mg. calcium, 33 mg. phosphorus, 0.7 mg. iron, 8 mg. sodium, 406 mg. potassium, 2,280 I.U. vitamin A, 18 mg. vitamin C, 1.34 mg. niacin, and 0.12 mg. zinc.

THERAPEUTIC BENEFITS

Nancy Ann Summers of Polson, Montana told me the following story about her own success with nectarine juice back in 1981:

> "I was staying with my elderly grandmother and helping to take care of her. She was recovering from partial paralysis of her right side due to a recent stroke. One day she began experiencing a shaking or trembling all over her body. This worried me, so I took her to our family doctor.
>
> "After carefully checking her over and spending more than an hour with her, the doctor (a woman also) announced to me: 'Well, it appears that your grandmother is suffering from spasmus agitans. This is a neurological syndrome often resulting from a deficiency of the neurotransmitter dopamine. This is a consequence of certain degenerative, vascular, or inflammatory changes in the basal ganglia.'
>
> "I stood there with my mouth open, trying hard with my high school education, to figure out just what in the heck she meant by all of this gobbley-gook jabber. Finally, I went 'Huh?' and she replied, 'Your granny has Parkinson's disease,' and I went, 'Oh, I see.'
>
> "Believing in natural healing myself, I went to a retired naturopathic physician for some recommendations. He said that in several cases similar to my grandmother's he had put his patients on *fresh* nectarine juice every day, *provided* they did not have *any* blood sugar problems. I distinctly remember him emphasizing the word *fresh* over canned or bottled juice.
>
> "Knowing that grandma wasn't diabetic or hypoglycemic, I went ahead and ordered several cases of fresh nectarines from the Red Cooper farms in Alamo, Texas. I would then make her some fresh

nectarine juice, leaving the skin on them but taking out the stones. She got half a cup of this morning, noon, and night before her meals. In about three weeks I began to notice her condition improve and outside of five weeks her constant trembling had been reduced to an occasional quiver every now and then. I believe the juice did her a world of good."

Crohn's Disease. This autoimmune disorder principally affects many parts of the digestive tract. In turn, secretions from these organs can exacerbate the problem more. The abundance of carbohydrates or natural sugar complexes in nectarine juice help to minimize the situation by soothing inflammations in the ileum and colon.

Muscle Twitching. Twitching of the mouth, facial spasms, wrinkling of the forehead, and eye blinking most commonly characterize those with tics or habit spasms. Head shaking, shoulder shrugging or arm or leg moving are other symptoms. These strange involuntary movements are done to relieve tension. For those who've seen the "Pink Panther" movies, they will recall the frequent eye and facial twitchings of the fictional French police Inspector Dreyfus (expertly played by Herbert Lom) whenever he heard the name of Inspector Clouseau (with the late Peter Sellers in the title role of the accident prone, bumbling detective). Nectarine juice has been of some benefit for those who suffer from muscle twitching. It seems that the high amount of potassium satisfies body tissue enough so that the muscles become more relaxed.

METHOD OF PREPARATION

The best value for the money in shopping for nectarines is to look for those which are slightly bruised due to shipping and handling. They are ripe and ready to eat. Wash each nectarine with soap and water and cut away the bruised sections. Then remove the pit but leave the skin intact. Cut into halves for easier juicing. One and one-half nectarines make close to a half cup of juice. You may need to add a little water if juicing in a Vita-Mix to make a thinner juice.

NETTLES JUICE

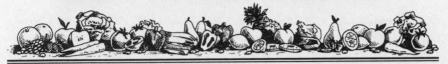

"First Aid for Hemorrhaging"

DESCRIPTION

This perennial (*Urtica dioica*) is most notable for its stinging qualities which disappear, however, after being slightly simmered. It is also one of the first single-stalked greens to appear in snowy regions in the springtime.

The stalks, the stems of the leaves, and the leaves themselves bristle with a fine stinging fuzz in which formic acid is a major irritant. (Formic acid, by the way, is the same irritant dispensed with the bite or sting of a red or black ant!) Therefore, it is best gathered with knife or scissors and disposable paper bags, with one's hands protected by impermeable leather, rubber, or plastic gloves. Indians, not having these, counteracted the resulting itch both with crushed green dock leaves and with the rusty feltlike sheaves of young ferns.

Slim, lengthy, branched, inconspicuous bunches of small verdant blossoms grow rather late in the summer in some localities, in angles between stalks and leaf stems.

NUTRITIONAL DATA

One-half cup of stinging nettle juice is a powerhouse of nutrition because of these essential minerals and vitamins: 167 mg. calcium, 86 mg. phosphorus, 3.2 mg. iron, 72 mg. sodium, 311 mg. potassium,

4,715 I.U. vitamin A, 57 mg. vitamin C, 91 mg. vitamin P (bioflavonoids), 112 mg. magnesium, and 7 mcg selenium.

THERAPEUTIC BENEFITS

Edith Yancey of Twin Falls, Idaho submitted this story to me awhile back concerning the use of nettle juice for first aid purposes:

"My husband is a scoutmaster. He took his troop of boys on an extended hike into the mountains. One of them slipped and fell and cut himself pretty badly on a sharp rock. A tourniquet was applied to slow the bleeding.

"Being something of a plant expert himself, he decided to hunt around for some stinging nettle, knowing that it would help with the wound. Finding a clump of it on a steep moist embankment, he put on some thick work gloves he had with him, and proceeded to pick a quantity of it.

"Taking what he had gathered back to camp with him, he laid the nettle on a cutting board and chopped it into smaller pieces. He then took one of the scout's tan neckerchiefs, soaked it in some water and wrung it half-way. He arranged the chopped nettle in a little mound in the center of the cloth, then folded the corners in and turned it upside down.

"He then took the blunt hammer-end of a hatchet some of the boys used to split branches with for fire wood and began beating the top of the folded neckerchief a number of times. The boy, whose neckerchief it was, moaned about the stain it would leave and the heck he would catch from his mom for this, but my husband paid no attention to this at all.

"He then unfolded the neckerchief and took the wet, juicy, pulpy green mass and applied it directly over the injured scout's wound and gave him explicit instructions to hold it there until the bleeding stopped. I can tell you that everyone was pretty amazed at how quickly the bleeding stopped—almost within minutes, it seemed!"

Cardiac Edema, Chronic Swelling, Trauma and Venous Insufficiency. German doctors have always been light years ahead of American physicians in the use of natural substances to complement the synthetic pharmaceuticals available to them. The late physician,

Rudolf Fritz Weiss, M.D. kept updating one of the most popular works ever written on natural medicine, his classic *Lehrbuch der Phytotherapie*. His last (6th) edition came out in 1985 (Stuttgart: Hippokrates Verlag GmbH) shortly before his death at an advanced age. Here is the English translation of part of the medical information he gave doctors relative to nettle juice and the conditions cited above. "Kirchhoff has noted that a pure expressed juice made from fresh nettles (Shcoenenberger) has a definite diuretic effect in cases of cardiac edema and venous insufficiency. Recent medical data has made us more cautious in the use of digitalis (foxglove) for decompensated heart conditions, and in mild to medium-severe cases one will first try to manage with gentle diuretic therapy. Here nettle juice is definitely useful. It has the great advantage of being well tolerated and completely safe, as distinct from the thiazides that are so widely used. Nettle juice can fill a gap in those situations, because it can be given well before the need arises for one of the very powerful synthetic diuretics. The same applies to other indications such as venous insufficiency, and also with edema of other origin, i.e., chronic swelling following traumatic injuries." (None of my readers may know this, but I speak and write German.)

METHOD OF PREPARATION

Pick and wash nettle leaves with gloved hands. Then juice in the same way as you would for spinach, romaine lettuce, or similar leafy greens. If intended for internal purposes, only a small amount (about one-half cup) of nettle juice needs to be consumed at one time. When external applications are desired, soak clean cloth or double-layered gauze material in the fresh juice, gently squeeze out excess liquid, and put directly on the surface of the skin.

OKRA JUICE

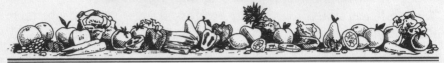

"An Alternative to Blood Transfusions"

DESCRIPTION

Okra (*Hibiscus esculentus*) sometimes goes by the name of gumbo, especially down New Orleans way. This tall, handsome, tropical annual is believed to have originated somewhere in Ethiopia, but found great popularity with the people of the Nile River Valley. Okra has a much-branched coarse stem that grows to a height of three feet and produces large-petaled flowers and long, slender, pointed seed pods. The pods are picked green and cooked to make a gumbo or mucilaginous body for thickening certain dishes. They are also cut up for soups. The ripe seeds have been used as a substitute for cofffee.

Although okra looks somewhat like a legume, it is a member of the Hibiscus family and is closely related to cotton. It thrives in areas that have long, hot, not too wet summers. Okra may be boiled, baked, or fried, but it is mainly used in Creole cooking. In the South, fried okra is a prized delicacy, and in New Orleans gumbo recipes, okra is combined with chicken or shellfish.

When okra is cooked, it becomes rather slippery, and, for this reason, it seems that much of the rest of the country has an apparent antipathy for it. Yet, this pretty pod has a delicious, artichoke-like flavor and a meaty bite. Okra's peak season is June through August.

Be sure to select firm, rich green unblemished pods that are less than three inches long. The baby whole frozen okra is far superior to the frozen cut okra.

NUTRITIONAL DATA

One cup of okra (equal to 100 grams by weight) yields: 92 mg. calcium, 51 mg. phosphorus, 0.6 mg. iron, 3 mg. sodium, 249 mg. potassium, 520 I.U. vitamin A, 1 mg. niacin, 31 mg. vitamin C, 38 mg. magnesium, 14 mg. sulphur, and trace amounts of copper, manganese, and iodine.

The seeds of okra, while impossible to juice, have been discovered to be a valuable source of protein. According to the *Journal of Agricultural and Food Chemistry* (23:1204–6, 1975), "the amino acid composition of okra seed was found to be similar to that of soybeans."

THERAPEUTIC BENEFITS

For several decades now, medical researchers around the world have been trying to find an ideal blood substitute for transfusion purposes. The reasons for this are varied, but legitimate. For one thing, members of certain religions cannot take blood transfusions on religious grounds. For another, some of today's available blood from various blood banks around the world is believed to be contaminated with the HIV virus, which is known to cause AIDS. A third reason has been the ongoing shortage of particular types of blood.

An inventory of scientific reports in the *Cumulated Index Medicus* for the years 1980-1982, showed that medical researchers in the United States, Australia, Japan, China, and the Soviet Union were all conducting experiments on different materials in hopes of finding effective blood substitutes. While the ultimate goal of developing a perfect "artificial blood" still remains in the future, work accomplished in the past has turned up some surprising things.

For instance, the Russians came up with a plant-derived substance which they called "rheogluman." This multifunctional blood substitute was used as a temporary plasma expander in the complex transfusion therapy of peritonitis caused by acute appendicitis (*Klin.*

Khir. 11:47–9, Nov. 1980). An even closer approach was made in 1988 by Australian medical researchers working out of the Commonwealth Scientific and Industrial Research Organization in Canberra. They discovered the presence of hemoglobin, the oxygen-carrying component in blood, in some plants. It led them to speculate that "hemoglobin genes might be present in all plants" (*Science News* 133:39, January 16, 1988).

For our purposes, the most intriguing material successfully tested thus far as a potential blood volume expander in some countries, has been okra pods. I first became interested in this vegetable when my friend, Dr. James Duke, who then worked for the USDA's Germplasm Resource Lab in Beltsville, Maryland, sent me some photocopied pages from *The Wealth of India* (New Delhi: Council of Scientific & Industrial Research, 1959, 5:86–87) on okra. It explained, in part, how a mucilaginous preparation from the pods had been successfully used as a plasma replacement. Mongrel dogs had been bled to a state of shock and then injected with a transfusion mixture of okra pod mucilage and a very small quantity of the animals' own blood. Every dog "recovered completely when transfused with the preparation…"

This led me to seriously consider okra as a potential blood plasma expander. I had a chance to test this theory out a few years ago while I was in Charleston, South Carolina doing some radio-TV appearances and public lectures for Books, Herbs, and Spices, a properous health food emporium. An African-American woman of about 41 years of age, who gave her first name as Ida, explained to me that she was shortly scheduled to go into surgery for a hysterectomy. Her doctors were facing the dilemma of finding enough blood for the necessary transfusion she would need, because of her rare blood type. She said an analysis of some of her blood had shown she was of the Sutter blood group with the Js[a] antigen being the dominating trait. Her physicians had told her that this only occurs in about 19 percent of the American black population and is extremely rare in other minority groups. If a donor of the same comparable blood type couldn't be found soon, they would be forced to postpone her operation indefinitely.

Her question, therefore, didn't have to do with herbs for the problems for which she was having the hysterectomy, but rather if there was something that would help increase her blood supply in the event a suitable donor of matching blood type couldn't be found in time. I had to admit to her that in all my years of professional health expertise, I had never been confronted with a question like this.

After pondering the matter over in my mind for a few minutes, I advised her, first of all, to donate some of her own blood weeks in advance of the operation, and then to have the surgery rescheduled for a month later. The inspiration also came to me, based in part on the Indian report, to tell her to start drinking okra juice (one cup) each day with a meal for several weeks up to the time of her surgery, and to resume the same regimen after her discharge from the hospital.

"You'll discover," I added, "that by doing this, your body won't require as much extra blood as you might think. Your doctors will only need to give you a very small amount of your own blood, with plenty to spare, because the okra juice which has been circulating around in your blood plasma will act as a substitute of sorts, for what would have been extra blood transfused into your system." She gave me an odd look, due to the strange information I had just imparted to her. I, too, felt a little bit awkward by what I had just said, but felt comfortable enough to know that it would work. "At least okra juice is nutritious enough that it can only help you," I stated. This reassurance gave her more confidence in my advice.

I happened to remember the incident a few months later, and called her on the telephone to inquire of the results. She was delighted and pleased to speak with me again. Ida confirmed that everything I had told her happened just as I said it would. After the first week, she decided, on her own, to increase her daily allotment of okra juice to two cups. She said her doctors were amazed that she required *so little* of her own previously donated blood during surgery. They couldn't understand the reason for this. I asked her exactly how much she required, she guessed that it was less than half a pint!

The November, 1977 issue of *Prevention* health magazine quoted Dwight McKee, M.D. as saying that he used a combination of celery and okra juices and whey for treating patients suffering from stomach ulcers and rheumatoid arthritis.

Autoimmune Diseases.   These are disorders in which the immune system attacks the body's own tissues. Normally, the immune system doesn't react against the body's cell and proteins. In autoimmunity, the immune system's tolerance is disturbed, and it releases autoantibodies that attack normal body cells. An autoimmune response causes varying degrees of tissue damage. It affects women more frequently than men. Cooked okra and okra juice are of considerable value in such instances. While okra can't stop the problem, it can definitely alleviate much of the joint pain, muscle weakness, malaise, and fatigue common to such disorders. It does this via its rich protein and trace elements contents.

Gastrointestinal/Glandular Inflammations. These are quite common occurrences in autoimmune responses. Okra has unique carbohydrate (sugar)-protein (amino acid) complexes, which enter the circulating blood plasma and go directly to specific sites of inflammation where they provide nourishing relief to swollen tissue and glands.

METHOD OF PREPARATION

Fresh okra pods make the best juice. They are springy and resilient and show no signs of surface discoloration. But be forewarned that they are *highly* perishable and ought to be promptly used after purchase. Wash the pods under running water before paring away the tough stem end and cap, being careful, however, not to puncture the pod itself. Then lightly steam them for no more than four minutes. Afterwards, place both the whole pods and their cooking liquid into a Vita-Mix for about one and one-half minutes to make a delicious juice out of them. A little extra water may need to be added to dilute the thickness of the juice.

The washed pods can be run through a juicer without removing their stems and caps and without any pre-cooking. Either way, the juice will have a solid alkaline taste to it, reminiscent of artichoke juice.

OLIVE JUICE

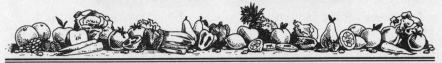

"Softening Agent for Skin Tissue"

DESCRIPTION

Olives (*Olea europaea*) are about as ancient as the first civilizations which grew them. In the Old Testament story of Noah, it was an olive twig that the dove returned to the Ark to give word that the great Flood was starting to recede. One Biblical scholar has asserted that no tree is more closely associated with the history of mankind and the development of civilization than is the olive.

Olives are often mentioned in old Greek and Roman writings, as well as in the Bible, and they were used in ancient Egypt 4,000 years ago. Today the tree has been introduced to many different parts of the globe where there is a suitable Mediterranean climate. Olive trees, many of them gnarled with extreme age, grow profusely everywhere around the Mediterranean — except Egypt — and also at the eastern end of the Black Sea. Their beautiful silvery olive-green foliage is the characteristic covering of the hillsides. Olives are evergreens. In springtime they are covered with insignificant flowers which drip gum all over any car carelessly parked beneath. Later in the year the trees form green berries which turn black or very dark purple as they ripen.

There are many varieties of olive differing in size, color, oil content, and flavor. Flavor is also greatly influenced by locality, but the flavor of the olives and of the oil which is expressed from them has no direct connection with size or appearance. The best flavored olives are often small and unimpressive to look at, and often grow in rough looking locations in remote mountain valleys.

Crude olives are intensely bitter and quite inedible; the bitterness has to be washed off with several changes of water and also gradually disappears when olives have been pickled for some months in brine.

Green olives are gathered unripe: black olives are ripe olives. The olives, tidily packed in bottles, which people are used to in the United States, give no indication of the huge variety sold loose in the stalls of any big Mediterranean market—especially in Spain. Olives may be bought stoned and stuffed with slivers of red sweet pepper, almonds or anchovy; flavored with thyme, garlic, fennel, and other herbs; and crushed, pickled or fermented. When these methods are superimposed on various species, the permutations are endless. In these foreign markets you not only can, but are expected to taste the wares before you buy them.

NUTRITIONAL DATA

Ten ripe olives yield the following nutrients: 40 mg. calcium, 8 mg. phosphorus, 0.8 mg. iron, 385 mg. sodium if pickled and just 4 mg. sodium if unpickled, 16 mg. potassium, and 30 mg. vitamin A. If pickled olives are to be used for juicing purposes, they should be soaked in cold water and rinsed several times to remove most of the excess sodium.

THERAPEUTIC BENEFITS

If one has the good fortune to ever visit the peninsula of Methana in the Peloponnesus in southern Greece, there will be found "the queen of all trees" in great and grand abundance. Villagers everywhere store plenty of olive oil, which they use for cooking and baking purposes. It was also something of a curiousity to notice that many of the older women still retain a very youthful quality to their skin. By contrast, American women of the same ages, 45 to 75 years old, are fighting back wrinkles with everything they can.

I learned the "secret" in the town of Argos. There, Maria Praisos, a middle-aged, short, rotund, and very jolly lady, demonstrated how she kept herself virtually wrinkle-free. She took the juice of green olives, which is extremely bitter but very astringent and rubbed it on her face, forehead, neck, throat, hands, wrists, and forearms, much as some men might splash after-shave lotion on themselves after shaving. She moved her fingers in quick circular motions and patted the skin with brisk slaps. The strong astringency of the olive juice apparently kept her skin tight enough so that there was nothing loose enough to sag or wrinkle. The daily intake of olive oil with different meals gave resiliency and suppleness.

Due to the extremely high sodium content in pickled olives, it isn't advisable to go drinking the juice on a regular basis. Because the juice of unripe olives is so nasty-tasting and unsettling to the system, no further uses beyond cosmetic purposes are recommended here.

Intestinal Parasites.   There are very few things which I've ever seen green or ripe olive juice used for. Most of the medicinal applications worldwide are for the oil. However, in parts of Indonesia, the bitter juice of the unripe olives has been successfully used in carefully measured doses for expelling worms from children and adults. I believe it's the nasty-tasting tannins in the juice, which has a remarkable "knock-out" effect on all types of intestinal parasites.

METHOD OF PREPARATION

If you are able to obtain green or unripe olives directly from the tree, then do so. Remove the stones and wash them. Run them through your juicer, adding a little water as necessary if the juice becomes too thick. Store in the refrigerator in a sealed plastic container and rub a little bit every morning on the skin. If using pickled olives, soak and rinse them several times to remove the excess salt. Then cut out the stones and juice. Some of this can be rubbed on the skin or else one-fourth cup taken internally, provided you don't have hypertension. A small residue of salt is bound to remain in the olives, even after several good rinsings. This may aggravate existing high blood pressure in those placed on sodium-restricted diets by their physicians.

Actually a combination of one-quarter pickled olive juice and three-quarters celery juice, rubbed on the skin in small amounts as well as taken internally, makes a good skin tonic. The secret here, though, is to *briskly* rub this liquid combination on to the skin with the fingertips. One table-spoonful of olive oil every other day, taken internally, doesn't hurt either.

By far the best application, however, is the green, unpickled olive juice used externally. This seems to work better than the other for preventing wrinkles.

PAPAYA-MANGO JUICES

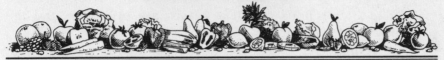

"Liquid Assistance for Hiatal Hernias"

DESCRIPTION

Papaya (*Carica papaya*) is an herbaceous, fast-growing, short-lived, palm-like plant that is native to tropical America and cultivated from the Mexican lowlands to Peru, Bolivia, and Brazil. Essentially, papayas grow like weeds throughout the tropical zones of the world. Some can get as big as footballs.

Hawaiian papayas are carefully tended and nourished. Almost all are of uniform size and are identical in appearance. Usually a light green in color when harvested, they color up to a golden yellow as they ripen, following the same changing color pattern as bananas. Just about all of the papayas sold in North America are grown in Hawaii and are shipped by air to the mainland and Canada.

The main Hawaiian variety is called Solo, but there is nothing solo about the way they grow. When I was in the Hawaiian Islands in late 1981, I saw hundreds of this kind on a single papaya tree. The Solo is a yellow-fleshed variety. There has also been an increased supply of an orange-pink-fleshed variety called the Sunrise. Both varieties are equal in flavor and texture and will ripen at room temperature.

Fully ripened papayas are golden yellow in color. When they are green they are not mature and lack the necessary flavor. The best way to prepare them for juicing purposes is to peel then cut them lengthwise, from stem to blossom end. Next scoop out the numerous black seeds. Then add a few drops of fresh lime or lemon juice to jazz up the rather bland but sweet flavor before running the fruit through your juicer. Ripe papaya juice will taste very similar to ripe cantaloupe juice.

Mango (*Mangifera indica*) is a tall tree with a broad, rounded top and clear, resinous sap. The leaves are evergreen and the pleasantly aromatic flowers are pink or yellowish in color and profuse in numbers. It is believed the mango originated in India and Myanmar (formerly Burma). To the people in the tropics, this tree plays a similar role to that of the apple tree in North America. Having been to parts of Indochina where it is not uncommon to sometimes see a huge mango tree fifty feet tall *and* wide in circumference, I have tasted vine-ripened mangos. With the possible exception of a ripe honeydew or perfectly ripe pineapple, I know of no other fruit that is so sweet or fragrant. In fact, if one isn't careful he or she is apt to "pig out" on these delicious mangos to the point of almost getting sick.

Mangoes come in assorted varieties, sizes, colors, and shapes. They can be as small as a hen's egg and weigh only a few ounces or be as large as an ostrich egg and weigh upwards close to four pounds.

Most mangoes have a fair-to-excellent flavor about them, but the one to avoid is a fairly flat, kidney-shaped, green-skinned mango with a red cheek, called an oro. With the exception of its flesh color there is really nothing golden about this variety. It is stringy, tastes like turpentine, and usually spots up and decays before it ripens. If you have ever had an experience with an awful mango, chances are it was with an oro. They are imported from Mexico because we don't know any better, and those who grow it south of the border sell it to us for its eyeball appeal and because it's the first variety to hit the market.

While there can be some dispute as to whether the mango is the world's sweetest fruit, there is no argument that it is the sloppiest. This fruit wasn't designed for dainty eating by any means. The combination of a very juicy flesh and a large, flat pit that isn't freestone makes it imperative that you either wear a bib or have lots of paper towels handy when you tackle a mango to eat.

In the tropics, where serving mangoes is a rule rather than an exception, they use silver mango forks with four long tines. A very ripe mango is skewered and the skin is scored with four lengthwise cuts. The skin is then peeled down like a banana and the fruit is eaten like an ice cream bar.

When I was in Thailand and Malaysia, I learned a trick about eating ripe mangoes without a lot of paper napkins. I would gently roll them on a table as you might do to soften a hard lemon. When the pulp was almost liquid, I made a small incision at the stem and sucked out the nectarlike pulp. This method I employed only with very ripe mangoes. The flavor is almost tutti-frutti, or a combination of very ripe peaches, apricots, and pineapples.

NUTRITIONAL DATA

One medium-sized ripe papaya contains the following nutrients: 61 mg. calcium, 49 mg. phosphorus, 0.9 mg. iron, 9 mg. sodium, 711 mg. potassium, 5,320 I.U. vitamin A, 170 mg. vitamin C, and 31 mg. magnesium. One mango yields the following minerals and vitamins: 23 mg. calcium, 30 mg. phosphorus, 0.9 mg. iron, 16 mg. sodium, 437 mg. potassium, 11,090 I.U. vitamin A, 81 mg. vitamin C, and 18 mg. magnesium.

THERAPEUTIC BENEFITS

Bob Lynnhaven of Columbia, South Carolina had been bothered with a hiatal hernia for a number of years. After every meal he would experience heartburn and sometimes severe pain behind the lower end of his breast bone. It became worse if he stooped over or laid down on the couch. At other times he would bring up small amounts of bitter greenish material.

He had already resorted to sleeping in a propped up position with pillows, consuming small meals frequently, and avoiding heavy work that required much stooping. He was still experiencing some misery. A friend told him to suck on some Rolaids, which gave him a little relief but not much.

Since Bob didn't have the time or patience or funds for a juice machine, I recommended bottled or canned papaya and mango juices. I instructed him to mix one-quarter mango juice with three-quarters papaya juice so they would equal a 6 oz. glass of liquid. He was to slowly sip this through a plastic straw after every 3 or 4 well-chewed bites of food were swallowed.

Bob sent me a "thank you" note some time later, saying that within days, "I was perfectly cured of my hiatal hernia, since following your advice."

Like the date-fig juice combination mentioned earlier in this book, the papaya-mango blend is helpful for a large number of different problems. Two things which make this blend so useful are the high amount of carbohydrates and enzymes in both fruits, that work together to promote healing within and without the body. This is especially true where swelling and inflammation, gastrointestinal difficulties, fever, and pain are concerned.

While papaya-mango juice won't solve every problem mentioned below, this combination should at least help to alleviate some of the suffering they cause. As with date-fig juice, the same *cautionary note* is again urged for those having blood-sugar problems (diabetes and hypoglycemia), allergies, or yeast infection (candidiasis). Because such fruits are high in natural sugar content, their use may need to be restricted under these conditions, so that existing symptoms aren't further aggravated.

Complexion Problems.   The early natives of the Caribbean always utilized the papaya for cosmetic purposes. Their remarkable complexions were attributed to the use of the ripe pulp as a skin soap. The juice of the same fruit pulp was used to get rid of freckles or wrinkles caused by the intense heat of the sun.

Dehydration.   Mango juice is frequently used in India, Malaysia, and the Philippines as a thirst-quenching agent to relieve dehydration.

Circulation (Poor).   Mango pulp *with* the juice promotes sluggish blood circulation. It is used in this capacity by folk healers in Vietnam, Thailand, and Malaysia.

Spleen/Liver Enlargements.   The milky juice from unripe papaya fruit was highly valued in India by Ayurvedic doctors for enlargements of the spleen and liver, author E. J. Waring noted in his book, *Remarks on The Uses of Some of the Bazaar Medicines and Common Medical Plants of India* (London: 1883; p. 118).

METHOD OF PREPARATION

Wash, peel and remove seeds and stones from a ripe papaya and mango. Next cut into small quarter sections and then run through your juice machine separately. Store in two different plastic containers with tight lids on them. When using, mix one-quarter of mango with three-fourths of papaya juice. Add a half teaspoonful lime juice for extra flavor and *sip* (don't drink) one cup per meal.

PARSLEY JUICE

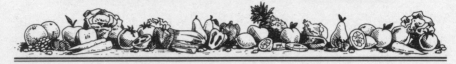

"Putting the Lid on Allergies Forever"

DESCRIPTION

Parsley (*Petroselinum hortense*) is a biennial that produces a bunch of finely divided and curly leaves the first year, highly valued for their aromatic-flavored properties. The leaves have the characteristic of neutralizing the pungent flavor of onion. The second year the seedstalk is sent up and produces a flat head of numerous small white flowers.

There are a number of types and varieties of parsley. The plain-leaved kind is not so common as the curled-leaf. The celery-leaved or Neapolitan is not generally grown in the United States. The fern-leaved variety is occasionally grown, while the Hamburg or turnip-rooted parsley variety is grown in market gardens near large cities.

NUTRITIONAL DATA

Ten sprigs of parsley contain: 20 mg. calcium, 6 mg. phosphorus, 0.6 mg. iron, 5 mg. sodium, 73 mg. potassium, 850 I.U. vitamin A, 17 mg. vitamin C, and 11 mg. magnesium.

THERAPEUTIC BENEFITS

People have asked me at different times, just how I manage to come up with so many food remedies for a wide variety of ailments. One of my responses has typically been, "Sometimes I'll try them out on myself first, and then if success is achieved I know they'll work on anybody. This is true with the use of parsley for allergies."

On the weekend of August 6–8, 1993, I was back in Kutztown, Pennsylvania, speaking at the local university there during the Pennsylvania Natural Living Convention. I stayed in one of the student dorms as hundreds of other visitors did. We took our meals, which were specially prepared for this event and made out of wholesome, organic foods, in the campus cafeteria.

During most of Friday and part of Saturday, I was in an older building which served as our exhibit hall. Either the mustiness of the place or someone's perfume or cologne or the trees and vegetation outside the open windows made me sneeze almost continuously. Not only was it extremely aggravating, but also terribly embarrassing. Here I was, a noted author and lecturer of alternative health topics, giving people advice on how to get well, and I couldn't even control whatever I was allergic to.

Saturday evening I joined some others by invitation and we all trooped down to the cafeteria. One of the things that immediately caught my attention in the serving line was a large stainless steel mixing bowl filled with washed, cut organic parsley. It was intended more for plate decoration, I believe, than anything else, because nearly everyone passing by took only a few sprigs.

For some strange reason, my brain connected with the visual image of this thing and immediately sent out a strong craving signal to my body which I could not resist. Those in front of and behind me looked on in humorous astonishment as I piled an empty plate full of these parsley sprigs. I poured some oil and vinegar dressing over the top of them and sprinkled some croutons on for good measure. It took me about half-an-hour of slow chewing to completely devour the entire plate of parsley; but something wonderful soon happened after all of this had digested—*my frequent sneezing completely stopped!* I still don't know what it was in the parsley that made this happen, only that the leafy herb is good for allergies!

Not long after this, I received a letter from one Alex Williamson in Scottsdale, Arizona. He had bought my book *Heinerman's Encyclopedia of Fruits, Vegetables & Herbs* (West Nyack, NY: Parker Publishing Co., 1988) and obtained my address from the back of it. He had been plagued with allergies for an unspecified period of time, had tried just about everything health food stores and various health books had to offer, and was getting very discouraged.

I wrote back and mentioned my own experience with the parsley in Pennsylvania. I suggested that he juice one bunch of parsley every day and drink it with his noon or evening meal. I said I believed it would help him where nothing else had. Well, he followed my recommendation and reported back within a month the results of the same. In three days his eyes stopped getting watery and itchy. In five days his sneezing ceased. Within ten days he felt "cured" and "like a new man again." Thereafter, he cut back to just three cups of parsley juice a week.

This is one of those instances where something I stumbled on to because of a sudden craving for it, in turn has helped others like Alex finally get a handle on their seemingly hopeless allergies.

Parsley is one fantastic juice for the restoration of health in the body. Because of its high mineral salts content, it quickly neutralizes the disease-causing acid condition of the blood and in its place introduces a very health-promoting alkalinity which does the body a lot of good.

Cellulitis.   This is an inflammation of cellular or connective tissue. It can also be a nonlocalized inflammation of the scalp but without the customary suppuration. In his outstanding treatise on medicinal plants, *Mon Herbier de Santé* (Paris: Laffont/Tchou, 1975), the renowned French herbalist Maurice Mességué, recommends that people suffering from cellulitis consume parsley voraciously. "You should gorge yourself on it, in salads, omelettes, in soups, as a juice, and with all of your meat dishes," he writes.

Mercury Poisoning.   With all of the recent attention given amalgam fillings, which dentists have routinely used, the public mind has been confronted with the very real dangers attending mercury poisoning. In his classic work, *Lehrbuck der Phytotherapie* (Stuttgart: Hippokrates Verlag GmbH, 1985; p. 237, 6th Ed.), the late Rudolf Fritz

Weiss, M.D. highly recommended parsley juice as an excellent way to get rid of toxic mercury residue from the body. He cautioned, however, that due to the high apiol content in parsley juice, it should be diluted in a second vegetable juice of some kind or with water, and taken in short doses with intervals of several weeks in between, where it's avoided.

Skin Problems.   Mességué praises the virtues of parsley juice for treating all manner of "skin affections." He believes that the reason parsley works so well in this regard is on account of the high mineral salts (especially potassium), which have an alkalinizing effect on acidic blood and a great flushing action on the kidneys.

METHOD OF PREPARATION

Wash a bunch of loose parsley by soaking it in a large pot or bowl in the sink and swishing it around with your hand. This causes any debris to fall to the bottom. Then adequately drain it before juicing in your Vita-Mix or similar machine. I am somewhat partial to the Vita-Mix, because it retains all of the nutritional goodness of the parsley. Nothing is lost and everything is used, whereas with other juicing machines there is always leftover pulp that no one seems to know quite what to do with it.

PARSNIP JUICE

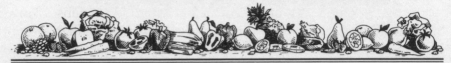

"Adding Lustre to Hair, Skin, and Nails"

DESCRIPTION

The parsnip (*Pastinaca sativa*) has sometimes been termed an "anemic carrot." Clearly this is a vegetable for particular palates, as its flavor doesn't attract people with very much enthusiasm, yet I can remember as a boy eating many kinds of soup, which my father used to fix for my brother and I, deliciously flavored with one or two cut up parsnips we bought at Speckart's Market down the street from where we lived in Provo, Utah.

This vegetable is grown for its long, slender, cream-colored root. It is a biennial and produces a much-branched seedstalk with the greenish-white, small, inconspicuous flowers arranged in a flat-topped head. The leaves are long and much divided. Parsnip is a native of Europe and of some ancient cultures too.

Parsnips are at their best flavor after they've been exposed to cold weather, and are at their poorest in midsummer. When stored in a cold, humid area or a refrigerator, they have an incredibly long shelf life. Parsnips go well with carrots in stews or soups.

Judge the quality of parsnips as you would carrots. Select those that are firm, crisp, and free from cracks. Medium-sized parsnips are preferable to those that are very small or very large. Avoid those that are discolored (brown instead of cream-colored) and those that are withered and limp.

NUTRITIONAL DATA

One large parsnip yields the following minerals and vitamins: 72 mg. calcium, 99 mg. phosphorus, 1 mg. iron, 13 mg. sodium, 606 mg. potassium, 50 I.U. vitamin A, 16 mg. vitamin C, and 40 mg. magnesium.

THERAPEUTIC BENEFITS

Joseph Cottrell, who lives just outside of Lane, South Carolina shared the following true episode with me some time ago:

> "My wife, you see, she's always been bothered with poor hair, skin, and nails. I mean, it's not like she has dandruff or is going bald. It's just that the ends of her hair keep splitting. I know that may sound crazy, but I don't know how to explain it better than that. And no matter what she does to her hair, it always seems to look the same sad and sorry mess everytime she fixes it up. I told her one time, I said, 'Honey, my bloodhound's coat looks better 'n your hair does.' I mean her no disrespect, but that's the truth I was telling her.
>
> "And you oughta see her fingernails. They keep splitting and sometimes got ridges and white spots on them. And her skin ain't in too good a shape either. Its always rough and coarse, never smooth like a lady's skin oughta be. You reckon you got something that may help her?"

Because he had included a phone number with his letter, I called him collect and inquired if he knew anything about parsnips. I knew he did when he replied, "You mean those funny-looking long white things in the store. Shoot, 'round here folks calls them 'sissy carrots' and won't have much to do with them. Excepting maybe for pig feed when the stores throw them out into the garbage."

I told him that his wife needed to be drinking some of this "sissy carrot" juice every day, mixed in with a little regular carrot juice or some leafy green juice of her choosing. This led me, of course, into another whole line of discussion about the importance of juicing and the best kind of machine for this. Not wanting to buy a juicer, he said he would look around to see if there was someone he knew who had one that he could temporarily borrow or rent. He must have found a juicer somewhere, because he was able to follow my instructions and have his wife drink a 6 oz glass of parsnip-carrot or parsnip-chlorophyll juice every day with one of her meals.

Several months later, I received a lovely note from Mrs. Cottrell, who thanked me for "working wonders" for her hair, skin, and nails. "My husband just can't get over how much those parsnips have helped," she added. "He figures that if our neighbor's pigs look good eating some of them every so often, then maybe it's probably gotta be good stuff for people, too."

Kidney Stones.   Renal calculi are hard, rock-like deposits that can develop anywhere in the urinary tract. They are made up of mineral and organic substances and range in size from a grain of sand to a golf ball. They develop when the salt and minerals contained in urine form clumps of crystals. When $\frac{1}{4}$ part of parsnip juice is combined with $\frac{3}{4}$ parts of any liquid chlorophyll and drunk on a regular basis, a number of these smaller crystals will begin to break up of their own accord and be discharged through urination. Only with larger stones of long duration will these juices not work. Kidney stones seem to be more common in those who eat a lot of meat and are heavy coffee or soda pop drinkers.

Overeating.   Eating too much or frequent snacking on high-calorie foods can lead to obesity. Compulsive or excessive food intake may be due to stress. Because of its high carbohydrate content, parsnip juice is able to satisfy some of these cravings. When one-third parsnip juice is mixed with two-thirds parts of carrot juice, the hunger pangs are soothed for up to four hours.

METHOD OF PREPARATION

A centrifugal or mastication juicer is the best machine for making parsnip juice. A juicer like the Vita-Mix, which I prefer over many others because of its versatility, is a bit limited when it comes to making juice out of a parsnip, but with a little patience and added water you can accomplish the job soon enough.

Wash and scrub one large parsnip with a wire vegetable brush. This way you won't need to peel it. Cut it into about 20 small pieces and slowly juice each of them. This should yield about one cup of juice. Parsnip juice tastes better if you mix it with either some carrot, beet, parsley, celery, zucchini, wheatgrass, or barley grass juice. Drink once a day with a meal.

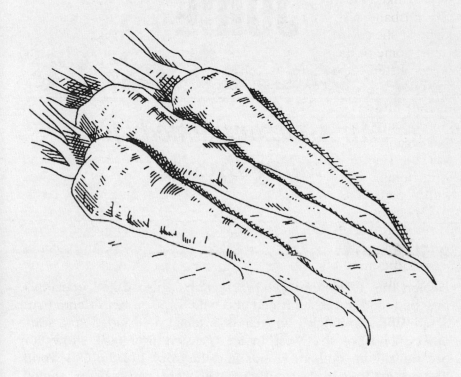

Parsnips

PASSION FRUIT JUICE

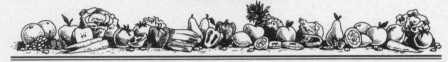

"An Amazon Remedy for Failing Eyesight"

DESCRIPTION

Passion fruit (*Passiflora quandrangularis*), also called granadilla, may be found in the cultivated and wild forms in both Central and South American jungles, as well as in Jamaica, Trinidad, and some other islands of the West Indies. Passion fruit also shows up occasionally in southern Florida and the tropics of the Old World. Passion fruit is an herbaceous vine, with stout, hairless, four-angled, winged stems, climbing by tendrils to almost sixteen feet in length. The leaves are alternate, on thick stems one-half to two inches long, bearing six glands and flanked by a pair of stipules which are broadly ovate and about 1½ inches long.

Passion fruit yields a very attractive blossom, called passion flower, which is marketed in some herbal markets in the U.S. and Canada. The flowers get up to five inches wide, are white, pinkish or purple on the inside, green or reddish green on the outside, and have white or pink-tinted petals that are usually one and one-half to two inches long. The flower crown is two-rowed, pinkish blue at the top, blue in the middle, and red-purple and white below. When the colors are taken all together, passion flowers present a rich, exotic, and strikingly beautiful pose.

Passion fruit is either pale green, frequently purple, or a beautiful combination of red and gold if it originates from New Zealand. It is about the size and shape of an ordinary large grade AA size hen's egg. In some ways it resembles a very small melon. Beneath the smooth inedible skin is a white, yellow, or pink flesh and a central cavity honeycombed with numerous seeds surrounded by purplish pink, juicy, acid pulp. The small seeds are nearly circular, flattened, and either black or purple-brown, and are a nuisance when eating the soft, ripe, fairly sweet fruit with a spoon.

Despite their rather sexy titles, neither passion fruit nor passion flower have any recognized aphrodisiac properties to them. To the contrary, they got their names from early Jesuit priests who came to South America several centuries ago and perceived the symbols of Christ's passion (the Crucifixion) in the various components of both the fruit and flower.

NUTRITIONAL DATA

One raw, purple passion fruit contains the following nutrients: 2 mg. calcium, 12 mg. phosphorus, 0.3 mg. iron, 5 mg. sodium, 63 mg. potassium, 130 I.U. vitamin A, 5 mg. vitamin C, and 5 mg. magnesium.

THERAPEUTIC BENEFITS

Most of the South American Indian tribes which were studied by ethnologists and other scientists in the late 19th and very early part of this century are no longer in existence. However, important data was gathered about their ways of life and incorporated into the scarce seven-volume massive work entitled *Handbook of South American Indians* (Washington, D.C.: U.S. Government Printing Office, 1946–59). The more recent work, *The Healing Forest: Medicinal and Toxic Plants of the Northwest Amazonia* (Portland, OR: Dioscorides Press, 1990) brings together additional data collected by a leading ethnobotanist and phytochemist on many of the plants previously used by many South American tribes. It is from both of these sources that the following information was obtained.

In the vast area of the Amazon Basin situated in Eastern Bolivia and Northeastern Brazil, resided the Chama and Macuna tribes. At the turn of the century there were just a few hundred members of both tribes still around. Besides utilizing the large abundance of tropical fruits growing in the wild, the Chama and Macuna also grew passion fruit, tomatoes, watermelons, pumpkins of several varieties, yams, taro, and beans.

When fully ripened on the vine, the passion fruit was picked, peeled, and the seeds removed. The soft flesh and juice was then put into a small wooden trough, which had been previously carved out of a section of log. A club-like stick with an enlarged rounded end was used to pound the fruit to a watery pulp. The juicy pulp was poured into another wooden bowl and then given to some of the elderly tribes people to drink for improving their failing eyesight.

Some of the other Amazonian tribes and sub-tribes utilized the juice from the pounded passion fruit and the crushed flower buds to reduce eye inflammation, to cure conjunctivitis, and to sharpen visual abilities.

The question, of course, is, "Does a remedy from the remote Amazon work for someone living in the concrete jungles of, say New York City?" Minerva Pendergast, age 67, from the borough of Queens believes it does. She was one of those who stayed after my lecture Saturday afternoon, April 23, 1993 in the Georgian Room at the Ramada Hotel in Manhattan, where I had been invited by the New Life Expo. Like the scores of others who crowded around me outside in the hallway and at my exhibit for the next hour or so, she wanted to know what could be done for her dimming vision.

Because my theme had been on the natural medicines of Native Americans in the Western Hemisphere, many wondered if there were likely remedies from the different tribes I referred to, for their own individual problems. I recommended passion fruit juice for Mrs. Pendergast, and suggested she drink one cup each day with a meal. Since the fruits themselves are more difficult to obtain than the canned or bottled juice, I advised her to buy it already prepared.

Several markets in her area, specializing in exotic and unique produce like this, carried what she wanted. On July 3rd of the same year, I received a postcard from her, saying, "...Oh, Dr. Heinerman, the remedy seems to be working. I doubt I'll ever be able to lay my glasses aside permanently, but, at least, I don't need to get a stronger prescription change. The dimness seems to have stabilized." I offer this testimonial as evidence that a remedy once used by now extinct stone-age tribes in the Amazon jungle, still works just as well almost a century later with some of those living in a more sophisticated kind of jungle here in the United States.

Those with blood sugar problems need to be careful in their use of passion fruit on account of its high sugar content.

Cystitis.   This is an inflammation of the urinary bladder. It can cause burning or difficulty during urination, blood in the urine, pain, fever, and other symptoms. Cystitis is more common in women, but rare in men. It is due to a bacterial infection by *E.coli.* In many Guatemalan *mercados* I've found vendors who not only sell the ripe passion fruit, but in some instances have offered ready juice on the spot. They get this by running some of the mature fruit through an iron meat grinder clamped to their display table. The result is a thick slush of sorts due to the pulp and juice being mixed together. Local *curanderos* routinely recommend the pulpy drink to women for the relief of urinary inflammation.

Insomnia.   In Trinidad the locals sell a bottled form of straight passion fruit juice, which they claim has terrific soporific effects. Any doubts in the mind which the average tourist may have about this are, quite literally, put to rest after a bottle or two of the stuff has been freely guzzled on an empty stomach. The person is usually out "like a light" within half-an-hour or less, depending on how tired he or she happens to be at the time.

Sore Throat, Tonsillitis.   In the northeastern part of the Amazon jungle, which is situated in part of Colombia, the Kubeos have routinely administered the juice of ripe passion fruit to their children who suffer from chronic sore throats. When I first became aware of this in my extensive jungle travels to that part of the world, I started recommending it to mothers in the United States for treating cases of tonsillitis in their young kids. From the feedback I've gotten from some of the many health conventions I speak at, where such information has been freely dispensed, it seems to be a good cure for this.

METHOD OF PREPARATION

If raw passion fruits can be obtained, they should be peeled and all of the seeds scooped out before being juiced. When fully ripe, they yield to very little pressure and juice easily.

PEACH-PEAR JUICES

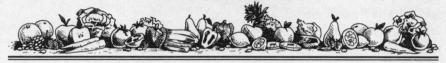

"An Effective Tonic for the Lungs"

DESCRIPTION

The peach (*Prunus persica*) is a low spreading, freely branching Chinese tree belonging to the rose family. It is quite cosmopolitan in cultivation in temperate areas of the earth. The tree yields lanceolate leaves and sessile flowers which are usually pink and appear on the naked twigs in the early spring. The typical peach season, depending on where you live in the lower 48 states, ranges from May to October.

The tree yields a drupe that is related to plums, nectarines, apricots, and almonds. This drupe is single-seeded and has a hard endocarp, a pulpy white or yellow mesocarp, and a thin downy epicarp, sometimes referred to as "peach fuzz." Peaches are grown in most states, but California and the South are still the largest producers. In fact, Georgia prides itself on being characterized as "The Peach State" and many communities have summer and fall events centered around peaches.

Fully ripened, juicy, peeled, and sliced peaches in fresh cream are one of nature's greatest taste delights. The color scheme they evoke in a bowl, with the golden yellow and ruby-tinged centers against a snowy white liquid background, makes for a truly beautiful contrast, which is probably where the expression "peaches-and-cream complexion" first originated.

The hundreds of varieties of peaches can be divided into two groups: the clingstones (also known as clings) and the freestones. There is a great difference in the flavor, texture, and succulence of clingstone and freestone peaches. Ninety-nine percent of the cling peaches are grown in California and sold to canners who put up tinned peaches and fruit cocktail; nearly all the freestone peaches are sold as fresh fruit.

If you've ever bitten into a California cling peach, you'll understand why they're sold to canneries. They are hard, rubbery, and without much liquid in them, and, quite frankly, are lousy for juicing. But cooking them in sugar syrup changes the undesirable texture and makes them quite palatable. However, after reading *how* commercial canneries remove the skins from them, I swore off eating any more canned peaches or fruit cocktail. Several articles in back issues of *Food Technology* and the *Journal of Food Science* explained how peaches are immersed for a few minutes in *lye* bath solutions so the skins can fall off quickly. Lye, of course, is strongly alkaline and always carries with it a "WARNING" label because it is so caustic and poisonous. Fruit salads just don't seem the same any more, unless I know the peaches in them are *fresh!*

When selecting peaches, choose the medium-sized ones, which can be every bit as flavorful as the larger and more expensive fruit. Try to get those which are unbruised. Let them set at room temperature for a few days to ripen properly.

The common pear (*Pyrus communis*) is one of the earliest cultivated fruit trees, both in its native Western Asia and in Europe. This member of the rose family and its fruit are similar to the closely related apple (considered by some botanists to be of the same genus) in characteristics and in method of cultivation, but the tree is somewhat less hardy and the fruit more perishable. Quince, another fruit, is closely allied to the pear.

Believed to have come from the foothills of Northern India and Afghanistan, the pear doesn't do well where the summers are too warm or the winters too cold. The West Coast and the Northwest have the ideal climate and altitude for growing this fruit, whose areas account for over 90% of our total crop. Like apples, pears must be harvested while still firm, long before they reach full maturity. Unlike peaches or mangoes, which are at their flavor best when allowed to tree-ripen, a tree-ripe pear will be unpleasantly soft and mushy to eat.

The Bartlett is the best eating and juicing pear. It made its debut in England in 1770 under the name of the Williams pear, but was renamed the Bartlett in 1820 when it was introduced to North America. This bell-shaped variety is the world's best-loved, best-selling, most fragrant, and handsome-looking pear.

When shopping for Bartletts, choose those that are light green in color rather than dark green. They are dark green when harvested. As they ripen they go from dark green to light green to pale yellow to golden yellow. When they are overripe, they turn brown. Beware of Bartletts which sport a red cheek. They may look pretty enough in a fruit tray or basket, but the plain green ones are tastier by far.

Wood from the pear tree is hard and dense and very expensive. It is sometimes used in specialty cabinetmaking. Some Oriental varieties of pear trees are grown as ornamentals.

NUTRITIONAL DATA

One whole, ripe peach contains the following essential nutrients: 14 mg. calcium, 29 mg. phosphorus, 0.8 mg. iron, 2 mg. sodium, 308 mg. potassium, 2,030 I.U. vitamin A, 1.5 mg. niacin, 11 mg. vitamin C, and 6 mg. magnesium. One whole, ripe pear contains: 13 mg. calcium, 18 mg. phosphorus, 0.5 mg. iron, 3 mg. sodium, 213 mg. potassium, 30 I.U. vitamin A, 7 mg. vitamin C, and 9 mg. magnesium.

THERAPEUTIC BENEFITS

Mattiedna Johnson, R.N. has been a nurse for well over half a century now. Seventy-five years of age in 1993, she lives in Cleveland, Ohio, but recalls an event involving peaches and their tree leaves which happened sixty-three years ago in Marianna, Arkansas, that forever changed her life.

She was out chopping cotton in the fields with her father, when her Aunt Mary came running to tell them that back at the house her mother was dying.

"I didn't know it then, but Mama had the galloping consumption and an abscess in her lungs," Mattiedna recalled. "I was just a twelve-year-old girl and hardly knew anything about doctoring." But, as if by instinct, she gathered some peachtree limbs for fans. "I noticed how cool the leaves felt, so I made a poultice from peach leaves which I smashed with a hammer and soaked in vinegar."

After the poultice was applied to her mother's chest, perspiration streamed off the sick woman's body. "I went 'round to Papa's side of the bed to pull her over to where the sheets were dry, and the abscess popped."

Figuring that if the cool peach leaves were helping her mother that much externally, Mattiedna decided to go outside and pick some of the ripened fruit which she believed would help her internally. Not bothering to wash or peel the fruit, she got her mother's vegetable grater, put it into a large pan, and proceeded to grate each peach on the finer part. The result was a lot of mushy pulp and juice, which was then poured into a glass and given to the sick woman to drink.

"I stayed with Mama for eighteen hours. I kept changing the poultice every so often and grating more ripe peaches for her to drink, until she had coughed the rest of it out."

"When the family doctor finally got there, he told Momma, 'it looks like a trained nurse took care of you.' I was just a girl then, but that's when I knew I wanted to be a nurse someday!"

Mattiedna was the only African-American to work on the medically-famous "Penicillin Project," where she helped isolate the mold and determine the diseases it would fight. She then became the only black nurse ever to be sent by the Methodist Board of Missions to Liberia, West Africa, where she served as a medical missionary.

Mattiedna claims a crucial discovery. "Working on the 'Penicillin Project,' which showed how cultured spores killed streptococcus hemolyticus," she noted, "my description of the spores' activity as 'Terrible Mice' led to the trade name of Terramycin." (This is the antibiotic drug developed by Pfizer pharmaceutical company in 1950, which ultimately wiped out scarlet fever.) (I am indebted to Kyle Roderick for some of this information.)

Pear juice will also do the same thing. I'm acquainted with an unusual case of tuberculosis, which was partially remedied with the assistance of this substance. A local street person, who goes by the name of Bernie, was diagnosed at a free clinic as having TB. He complained of the constant pain in his lungs everytime he coughed. I recommended to the doctor providing some basic care to Bernie, that he give his patient some pear juice to drink. The doctor went to the local food bank here in town and obtained ten or a dozen cans of whole pears. He gave them to Bernie, along with a can opener, and advised him to drink some of the syrupy juice every time he felt these stabbing pains.

Bernie did so until he had exhausted his supply and came back to the doctor for more cans of pears. He said it had helped to diminish the pain to the point where he could better tolerate his disease. Of course, Bernie's independent life style, stubborn ways, and poor eating habits don't allow him the opportunity to seek more serious treatment for an epidemic infection that will eventually kill him. But, at least, the pear juice appears to have helped limit his pain.

Fevers.   Peach and pear juices have a decidedly cooling effect upon the system in cases of mild-to-extreme fevers. In fact, when no other type of nourishment can be tolerated by the stomach, either of these are neutral enough to be given with good success.

Indigestion.   Where an acidic condition may prevail in the gut due to heavy consumption of greasy or spicy foods, or just simply overeating, a cup of either peach or pear juice, slowly sipped, will help to relieve some of the intestinal discomforts.

Morning/Motion Sickness.   Women who are pregnant or those subject to motion sickness while traveling, should have within reach some pear juice. It will calm even the worst case of "stomach heebie-jeebies," and seems to work a little better than peach juice does because it's not as sweet.

METHOD OF PREPARATION

Rinse a ripe peach and pear under running water. Cut the peach in half and remove the pit. Do not peel either fruit. Cut them into quarter sections and put into a Vita-Mix machine with one cup of cold water on medium speed for about 1 minute. Add a little more water if necessary. Makes about two cups of juice. Drink at *room temperature only*. Chilled juice isn't good for the body and will only harm already injured lungs.

A delightful health drink which is easy to prepare in a Vita-Mix, calls for one-fourth cups fresh peaches and pears (cut into small pieces), a dash of powdered ginger, and one-half cup sugarfree ginger ale. Mix on medium or high speed for twenty seconds. Some people like to add half a cup of ice cubes, which is okay to do if the lungs aren't inflammed in any way. This mixture yields about one and one-half cups of a health drink that's sweet, creamy, and refreshing to the palate.

For another great flavor treat, try mixing equal parts of pear and apple juice, with a dash of lime juice for a kicker. Now there's a nifty drink that will sensationalize your palate!

PEA JUICE

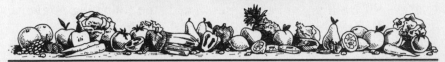

"Helps Dissolve Blood Clots"

DESCRIPTION

The common garden pea (*Pisum sativum* var. *arvense*) is a variety of the field pea. It is a trailing plant with oblong leaves and purple and white flowers. The fruit is a pod containing from four to ten seeds. The seeds may be smooth or wrinkled and green or cream colored. The varieties that are grown in the garden are sweeter than field peas and, in some cases, even the pods can be eaten. The field peas usually have a narrow and somewhat cylindrical pod, while the garden varieties have broad pods which are somewhat flattened. Peas are one of the most important vegetables from the standpoint of canning, ranking next to sweet corn in importance. It is one of the oldest vegetables in cultivation, having been grown in its native Egypt long before the Christian Era. As a green vegetable, however, it is not so important as snap beans.

When shopping for fresh peas the color is most important, and that color is green. Look for glossy, bright green, smooth-skinned pods. Check out the calyx—the remnant of the blossom at the stem end—and make sure it looks fresh and green. The pods should feel velvety. Reject those peas that are off-color (yellow) or dull and limp. Especially avoid those that feel very hard and have dry, rough pods. If they are in a mass display at your supermarket, open up a pod and examine and sample the peas. If they are sweet and tender, then

205

buy them. If they are hard or are starting to sprout, buy frozen or canned peas instead.

NUTRITIONAL DATA

One cup of fresh green garden peas yields the following nutrients: 38 mg. calcium, 168 mg. phosphorus, 2.8 mg. iron, 3 mg. sodium, 458 mg. potassium, 930 I.U. vitamin A, 4.2 mg. niacin, 39 mg. vitamin C, and 48 mg. magnesium.

THERAPEUTIC BENEFITS

Delbert Granger of New Albany, New York was having problems with his legs. Several smaller veins just beneath the skin on each leg were sore and swollen. In some ways they looked like hard, red cords. The overlying skin was always warm to his touch and splotched.

He consulted a physician, who looked at both legs carefully and then ran some tests. He then informed Delbert that he had superficial thrombophlebitis. "I had never heard of such a thing in my life," Delbert related to me later on. "I asked him, 'Hey, doc! What in the heck is that anyhow?'"

The doctor told Delbert that he must have banged his legs against something at the warehouse dock where he loaded and unloaded semi-trailers. Or he might have had a low-grade infection which led to this condition. What he had was an inflammation of a blood vessel in conjunction with a blood clot. Fortunately, for him none of the clots had broken away *yet* to circulate around in his bloodstream. When and if that happened, his condition could become more serious and risky.

The physician recommended bed rest at home with Delbert's legs elevated and warm compresses applied over the afflicted areas. He recommended that he take aspirin or some other anti-inflammatory drug which he could prescribe. "I didn't mind the bed rest or hot packs," Delbert said, "but I sure as the dickens didn't want him pumping me full of medications I had my doubts about, *including* aspirin!"

A friend of his wife's, who was told about his condition at their church one Sunday, recommended she try giving her husband some pea juice. "My wife's friend knew of a neighbor with similar problems and cleared it up in no time by juicing some garden peas. So we both figured, 'what the heck have we got to lose by trying this?'"

Within two weeks and after a return visit to his doctor, Delbert was pronounced free of any evidence of thrombophlebitis. "Though I don't have *that* problem any more," he joked with me, "I still have a problem pronouncing the dang thing, wouldn't you know?"

Celiac Disease. Symptoms of gluten-sensitive enteropathy (another name for it besides celiac disease and sprue) may become apparent in infancy when cereal is introduced or not show up until middle or late adulthood. Persistent diarrhea and being underweight are two common symptoms of it. Stools also tend to be typically bulky, light tan or gray, frothy and rancid smelling, and usually adhere to the bowl when the toilet is flushed. The stickiness is due to their high fat content. Adults with untreated sprue often excrete 30-40 grams of unabsorbed fat daily—about ten times the normal amount. Pea juice or pea soup (the heated juice) seems to alleviate these problems to quite an extent. The pulp included with the juice can help the intestines reabsorb food properly by mending the fingerlike projections called villi and the absorptive cells lining the small intestine, which have been damaged by gluten.

Irritable Bowel Syndrome. A groaning belly, a painfully distended abdomen, and spells of diarrhea and constipation are signs of irritable bowel syndrome (IBS). This is a perplexing long-term digestive disorder that affects about 15% of the entire U.S. population. Some cases of IBS are characterized not by diarrhea or constipation but by episodes of gut-wrenching pain that may not be related to meals or other external triggers. Bowel spasms are thought to account for this agony. Pea juice is of considerable value here, but *only* when it is *heated* and served *warm*. During the heating of the pea juice, a pinch each of powdered cardamom and ground ginger root should be added and stirred into the soup-to-be.

METHOD OF PREPARATION

Delbert and his wife used their Vita-Mix to juice the peas they picked fresh and ripe from their garden. "I put my cup of shelled peas in the two-liter container and set the left button to the variable position," Mrs. Granger told me. "I then turned the speed knob slowly up to number 3 position to sort of puree my peas before adding a little water. After it got to a runny consistency, I poured the liquid into a glass and gave it to him to drink with his lunch." She did this every day for the period of time stated until he was completely healed.

PEPPER
(GREEN BELL)
(See Chile Peppers Juice)

PERSIMMON JUICE

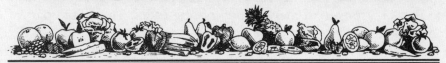

"Say 'Hasta la Vista' to Intestinal Parasites"

DESCRIPTION

The persimmon (*Diospyros virginiana*) is a native of ancient China and Japan and very popular in the Orient. It also happens to be a very unusual fruit. Not akin to any other kind of fresh fruit, it is related to the ebony tree. Just as ebony wood is highly prized for making furniture, persimmon wood is highly prized for making heads for golf clubs.

All of our commercially grown persimmons are produced in California because the fruit of the persimmon trees that grow wild in the Deep South are too small and fragile to have any commercial value. Persimmons have a rather short season; they are in the market from October to January and a few are brought in from Chile in the spring.

209

The Hachiya persimmon—one of two varieties grown in California (the other being the Fuyu)—is one of our most colorful and shapely fruits. It looks like a shiny, deep-orange-colored, acorn-shaped tomato. If allowed to fully ripen, there is no fresh fruit that is sweeter than a Hachiya. If it is eaten prior to reaching full ripeness, however, it is without question our worst-tasting fruit.

When buying persimmons, select those that are very firm and colorful. Don't buy those that have started to ripen up because they may be bruised. Allow the persimmon about three or four days to ripen at room temperature. When you are convinced that the persimmon is ripe enough to use, wait another day or two. When you are sure it is overripe and ready for the garbage can, then and *only then* will it be ready to be eaten. By that time the once beautiful persimmon will have shriveled and lost color. Unless the skin looks like a blister, it isn't quite ripe. The skin of the persimmon is similar to that of a tomato. It may or may not be eaten. The edible part of the fruit is seedless. Peel and juice it as a raw fruit.

Take it from one who knows, don't ever bite into a firm persimmon. I did so in mainland China back in 1980 and I can still recall the most horrible taste I believe I've ever experienced to date. It was worse than sampling an equal amount of alum. It is *so* astringent, some claim, that if enough is accidentally chewed or sucked on for any given time, it will plaster the most horrible frown imaginable on that unlucky person's face for days to come.

Let me share another little secret with you about the persimmon. If you take a baseball-hard, thoroughly unripe persimmon and stick it in your freezer and remove it later after it's frozen solid, it will, as if by magic, transform and become ripe, juicy, and not astringent at all when thawed out.

NUTRITIONAL DATA

One persimmon contains the following nutrients: 10 mg. calcium, 44 mg. phosphorus, 0.5 mg. iron, 10 mg. sodium, 2,992 mg. potassium, 4,550 I.U. vitamin A, 12.6 mg. folic acid, 13 mg. vitamin C, 15 mg. magnesium, and a high amount of fluoride as well as vitamin K.

It is this rich fluoride content which makes some African species

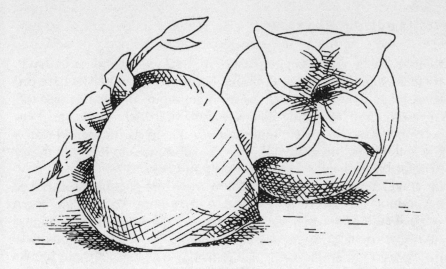

Persimmons

of persimmon so valuable as natural aids for dental hygiene. In various marketplaces in Nigeria, Ghana, and other countries on the continent, persimmon twigs and unripe fruit cut in half can usually be found. These "chewing sticks" as they are called, are first washed, then gnawed on the tip to macerate it so that the end is frayed and brushlike. The teeth are brushed very thoroughly, and care is taken to clean both the inside and the outside of the tooth surfaces. I've noticed that this procedure takes from five to ten minutes and often, the stick is sucked for several hours after brushing is completed. In fact, it's not an uncommon sight to see individuals going about their chores with the remainder of a chewing stick in the mouth.

The unripe fruit itself is cut in two, and one half of it is sometimes rubbed over the gums to prevent or correct pyorrhea and gingivitis. The unripe fruit also clears up cold sores, recurrent herpes and fever blisters on the lips and inside the mouth. Canker sores are also benefited by this peculiar treatment. All of these dental advantages are due mostly to the high natural fluoride content in the twigs and unripe persimmon fruit. This is the way we should be obtaining such an unpleasant-tasting trace element, instead of in the fluoridated water many Americans are forced to drink on a daily basis against their will and better judgment.

THERAPEUTIC BENEFITS

Different traditional herbalists and folk healers with whom I have visited in Nigeria, Senegal, Ethiopia, South Africa and elsewhere on the African continent, have been unanimous in their praise of persimmon fruit for getting rid of *any* type of intestinal parasites, but preferably when it is still somewhat *unripe*. In its unripened state, they insist, there are more nasty-tasting substances to help kill these harmful parasites than when it's sweet and ripe.

Take, for instance, an herbalist by the name of M'buki Henrique of Angola, who is what they call *Aladuras* in the Yoruba language or *Igbeuku* in the Bendel State area of Nigeria. He combines traditional herbalism with spiritual healing. He routinely goes out and collects different medicinal plants, berries, fruits, and roots growing near his private hospital. During his session with a patient, he will engage in praying after administering his vegetable or fruit remedy in order to induce a state of relaxation in the other person. In this capacity then he functions not only as an herbal doctor but also as a priest in faith-healing.

I watched as he administered a small wooden bowl of extremely bitter juice from two well-pounded persimmons to a young boy who's awfully distended stomach indicated a severe intestinal parasite problem. He said that within hours the awful juice would begin its work and drive out the worms causing his young patient so much pain and trouble. Coming back that way a few days later, my colleagues and I dropped in on M'buki and inquired about his young patient. He took us some distance to a row of houses in the village we were in and called out the lad's name. The boy who came over, we all noticed, had a fairly normal abdomen by now and was feeling first-rate and happy. This was the results of the unripe persimmon juice we were told.

Cuts.   Minor cuts are common when working around sharp instruments. They also can result from shaving in a hurry. Persimmon juice is the ideal astringent to dab onto the skin to stop minor bleeding. The best way to do it is to soak a cotton ball with the juice and then hold on the cut until bleeding ceases.

Hemorrhoids.   Piles (their common name) are nothing more than varicose veins within the anal area. They are similar to the twisted and swollen veins visible on some people's legs, especially in older women who have had several children. Rectal bleeding, rectal pain, itching and swelling are common symptoms.

Loose Teeth. Sometimes individual teeth may become slightly loose in the mouth due to a dental disorder, a nutrient deficiency, general malaise, or a sudden blow to the jaw. Persimmon juice is extremely astringent, meaning that it can cause a strong contraction or narrowing of the tissue to which it is applied. Saturate one or two cotton balls with persimmon juice and place them around the loose tooth and keep them there for awhile. Repeat the process frequently throughout the day for several days, or until the gum tissue has firmly secured the tooth in place again. Bleeding gums can also be treated by rubbing a cotton ball soaked in persimmon juice across them every day several times.

Varicose Veins. These are blood vessels that have become swollen and twisted because of an impairment of the internal valves that normally assume proper blood flow. Varicose veins most commonly develop in the lower legs. While persimmon juice is limited to what it can do here, it nevertheless offers women some hope for this ugly problem. There are three different types of valved veins located in the legs: deep veins embedded in muscles; superficial veins, which are just under the skin; and perforated veins, whose valves permit blood flow from superficial to deep veins. At the time that bulging starts to occur in the superficial veins, a woman should make a habit of rubbing several cotton balls soaked with persimmon juice on the backs of her legs every day in order to prevent the problem from becoming more severe.

METHOD OF PREPARATION

After ripening some persimmons for about five days at room temperature, they are then ready for use as medicine but, most definitely, not as a food treat to be enjoyed. They will, however, be less acrid than if they were to be used from the store without letting them set a few days.

   If the juice is simply unbearable to take straight, it can be mixed with an equal amount of apple juice or apple cider and swallowed that way. I recommend half a cup of juice on an empty stomach morning and night until the parasites have been totally cleared out of the intestinal tract.

PINEAPPLE JUICE

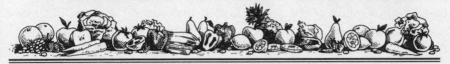

"Dissolving a Gastric Food Ball"

DESCRIPTION

The cultivated pineapple (*Ananas sativa*) produces a spiny, sweet, and juicy fruit that is believed to have originated in Brazil. It is now grown commercially in all tropical areas with a similar climate and soil. Hawaii, Taiwan, the Philippines, Mexico, and Central America are major producing centers.

The pineapple is highly prized as both a fresh and a canned fruit and canned pineapple juice is very popular. The Hawaiians were the first to can pineapples, which used to be their top industry before the advent of the jet age; now tourism ranks as number one. Today, much of our canned pineapple is processed in Taiwan and the Philippines due to the much lower labor costs in the Far East.

There are several varieties of pineapple. Those grown in Hawaii and most of those grown in Mexico and Central America are of a variety called the smooth cayenne. Those grown in Cuba and Puerto Rico are usually of the red Spanish variety. All varieties of pineapple are sweet and juicy if allowed to ripen fully before being harvested. Once the fruit is severed from the plant, it ripens no further. If picked after having reached full maturity and rushed to market without exposure to excess heat or chill, the pineapples will have a high sugar content and a juicy texture. If picked when immature, they will

215

be woody in texture and not very sweet. If they have been chilled, they will cut black. If they have been overheated in transit, they will be very soft and possibly have spots of decay.

While the pineapple is native to Latin America, it didn't reach flavor peak until it was transplanted to Hawaii. The pineapple thrives in Hawaii's ideal climate and great volcanic soil. Pineapples from Hawaii with green shells are picked at maximum ripeness, but I've noticed that those which have a trace of gold or orange color are much sweeter and juicier. The flesh of a fully ripe pineapple will appear to be glossy and wet. This is a plus and not a minus. It is a sign of high sugar content and full ripeness.

Refrigerators are a lousy place to store pineapples. The fruit should never be stored where the temperature is below 50° F. or it may cut black.

A compound derived from pineapple, bromelain, is used as an anti-inflammatory. This special enzyme, like the papain in papaya fruit, also is a key ingredient in meat tenderizer, and helps to digest food.

There are 1,500 species in 65 general categories in the Bromeliaceae or pineapple family. The well-recognized Spanish moss, which I've seen hanging from the old trees in downtown Savannah, Georgia, is a member of this family.

NUTRITIONAL DATA

One slice of raw pineapple contains the following nutrients: 14 mg. calcium, 7 mg. phosphorus, 0.4 mg. iron, 1 mg. sodium, 123 mg. potassium, 60 I.U. vitamin A, 14 mg. vitamin C, and 34 mg. magnesium. Some tocopherols (vitamin E components) have been reported also.

THERAPEUTIC BENEFITS

A type of ball which forms in the stomachs of some people following gastrointestinal surgery is called a phytobezoar. This is basically a gastric concentration formed of vegetable fibers, with the seeds and skins of fruits, and sometimes starch granules and fat globules.

Such a food ball forms after stomach surgery and decreases the amount of gastric juices secreted by the digestive tract. Further risk is enhanced by inadequate chewing of food and excessive consumption of fibrous fruits and vegetables.

The reduced contractility of the gastric remnant limits the amount of fiber that can freely pass into the intestine. Cellulose fibers that fail to pass then become entangled in a ball, which causes low-grade gastritis and the outpouring of a thick, tenacious mucus capable of binding additional fiber. In this manner a phytobezoar is formed.

The usual medical treatment for this has been gastrotomy, wherein an incision is made into the abdomen so the food ball can be lifted out with instruments. However, an interesting report published in the "correspondence section" of the *Journal of the American Medical Association* (236:1578) for October 4, 1976 revealed that there is a much safer, noninvasive way for coping with this problem.

A physician and registered dietitian working out of the Tufts-New England Medical Center in Boston reported that a 57-year-old woman, who had previously undergone surgery for a gastric ulcer, "sought to lose weight with a low-calorie diet containing increased amounts of fruits and vegetables." Several months later she began experiencing "frequent episodes of vomiting and postprandial epigastric distress." A stomach x-ray "showed an 8x13-centimeter bezoar." She was immediately placed on a low-fiber diet.

The unidentified female attempted to dissolve her phytobezoar by ingesting papain in the form of Adolph's Meat Tenderizer, but she quickly gave up that idea after "excessive burning discomfort made her stop within two days." She then asked her doctors about the possibility of taking bromelain instead. Doctors instructed her to drink about ten fluid ounces of *fresh* pineapple juice three times a day, half-an-hour before each meal. (This was slightly more than three full-sized drinking glasses of juice.)

JAMA reported the incredible results which followed this simple juice therapy in these terms:

> "Eight weeks later roentgenograms showed the bezoar to be half its former size, and her symptoms had improved substantially. Five weeks later the bezoar had completely disappeared. To prevent recurrence, the patient continues to take two 120 ml of the juice each day and is asymptomatic."

The enzyme bromelain dissolved the mucus "glue" and allowed the woman's ball to unravel by itself.

Enzyme Dysfunction.   An enzyme is a protein, secreted by cells, that acts as a catalyst to induce chemical changes in other substances, itself remaining apparently unchanged by the process. When there is any disturbance of normal enzyme function (including a genetic deficiency of key enzymes),this condition is called enzymopathy; but to keep it simple I've designated it merely as "enzyme dysfunction." Several tropical fruit juices are rich in specific enzymes: pineapple, which contains bromelain; and papaya, which contains papain. Both are extremely useful in the digestive tract to help break down animal and plant proteins, as well as perform certain pain-relieving functions within the body. In different parts of the text, I've reminded readers to *never* mix fruit and vegetable juices together, because they are generally incompatible with each other in terms of digestion. However, there may be an exception to this rule in that pineapple has frequently been used as a secondary juice for something else. I'm reminded of the wonderful story shared earlier by the Merritts of Salt Lake City under the KALE-COLLARDS entries. They prefer mixing some pineapple juice with these two vegetable juices to improve the flavor and help them digest better. I know that many juice lovers enjoy blending equal parts of carrot and pineapple together because of the great taste they provide. I might add, though, that this combination does create some minor intestinal gas problems for a few individuals, which gets back to my initial reason for *not* encouraging this, because of their digestive incompatibility. Still, though, I'm inclined to think that where specific enzyme action is needed with certain foods or juices, then it may be practical to combine a little pineapple or papaya with a vegetable drink.

METHOD OF PREPARATION

Previous information has provided some basic guidelines for selecting a ripe imported pineapple. Another way to tell, according to what an old Hawaiian told me some years ago in Laie, is to hold the fruit up close to your nose and carefully smell it. A ripe pineapple, he insisted, will smell "sweet" or have a hint of a sweet aroma about it, whereas an unripened one won't.

One piece of pineapple makes nearly a cup of juice. *Those suffering from diabetes or hypoglycemia* should exercise caution and use wisdom here. Because of the high sugar content in a ripe fruit, such individuals may need to pass on this particular juice altogether.

PLUM-PRUNE JUICES

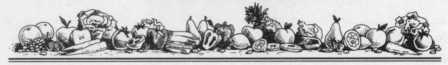

"Moving Experiences for Constipation"

DESCRIPTION

The terms plum and prune always cause some confusion, possibly because the Latin word for plum is *prunus*. (The genus *Prunus* is of the Rosaceae or rose family.) Botanically there is no difference between a plum and a prune. Originally in the English language, the words plum and prune were used as synonyms. Today, however, to make things easier, the Japanese varieties are called plums and the European varieties are called fresh prunes. The sun-dried fruit are also termed prunes.

The plum is a drupe and is related to the peach, nectarine, apricot, and almonds. Plums come in assorted sizes, shapes, skin colors, and even flesh colors. Some varieties are slightly larger than a marble, others are much larger than a jumbo egg. They can be either round or oval in shape. There is a wide range of skin colors: green, yellow, orange, purple, every shade of red, and black. Most plums have a yellow-colored flesh, but a few varieties have a red flesh. Most are clingstone, but several are freestone.

The European varieties are usually, but not necessarily, freestone. They all have yellow flesh, but the thing that sets them apart is that they always have a purple skin (sometimes it looks almost blue if it has a lot of bloom).

The Japanese plums come in a wide range of colors but never have the telltale purple skin color. Most varieties are also yellow in flesh, but some have a bright red flesh. Unlike the European plums, which for the most part are freestone, most, but not all, of the Japanese varieties are clingstone.

The Japanese plums are usually tastier and juicier than the European varieties. They are nearly always eaten out of hand or used as a fresh fruit, since they dissolve when cooked and are not suitable for drying in the sun to be marketed as dried fruit. The European plums have a milder flavor and a meatier texture. Some varieties are quite good when eaten out of hand, but most are at their best when cooked or baked. These are the only types that are sun-dried and sold as dried fruit.

When shopping for plums, select those that have good color, are at least medium-sized, and are unbruised. Remember to avoid buying the first plum varieties that arrive in market in early May. Wait until June for more flavorful, less costly varieties. Enjoy plums during the summer and early fall months. When the red-skinned varieties finally go out of season in mid-September, don't substitute with the large, attractive purple President plums, which lack flavor.

Nearly all the stone fruits (nectarines, peaches, and plums) should be purchased when firm and at high color, then allowed to ripen for a few days at room temperature. Once they attain a slight yield (or give) to gentle pressure, they should be stored in the refrigerator until used. Remember that slightly underripe is preferable to overripe. The one exception to this is the apricot. You can't have an apricot that is too ripe. They are at best flavor when the texture is almost fluid.

NUTRITIONAL DATA

One Japanese variety plum contains: 8 mg. calcium, 12 mg. phosphorus, 0.3 mg. iron, 1 mg. sodium, 112 mg. potassium, 160 I.U. vitamin A, and 4 mg. each vitamin C and magnesium. One prune yields the following nutrients: 3.3 mg. calcium, 5.1 mg. phosphorus,

0.25 mg. iron, 0.5 mg. sodium, 44.8 mg. potassium, 103 mg. vitamin A, 0.2 mg. vitamin C, and 3.8 mg. magnesium.

One cup of prune juice yields: 30 mg. calcium, 64 mg. phosphorus, 3.03 mg. iron, 11 mg. sodium, 706 mg. potassium, 9 I.U. vitamin A, 2 mg. niacin, 10.6 mg. vitamin C, and 36 mg. magnesium.

Annette M. Berry of East Hartford, Connecticut related the following in February, 1992:

> "A few years ago, I developed tendonitis in my right wrist, and my physician prescribed Motrin. Subsequent blood counts indicated that my blood count was dangerously low, indicating internal bleeding. Although the source of the bleeding was never found, it stopped when I was taken off the Motrin and iron pills were prescribed.

> "My blood count came up to normal, but I was still on iron pills. When I learned that iron pills were hard on the liver and that there were numerous natural plant sources for iron, I called my physician and told him I wanted to forego the iron pills and have three small glasses of prune juice a day with my meals. He agreed, but he wanted a blood test in six weeks to determine if the change would work.

> "After six weeks, the test showed that my blood count had remained just about the same. My doctor immediately determined that I no longer needed the iron pills and prescribed that I stay with the prune juice."

Annette's story shows the value of something like prune juice for natural iron supplementation, especially in women who seem to require more of this mineral than men do.

Prunes are also high in fiber. To get the same dietary fiber as a serving of six prunes, you'd have to eat four slices of whole wheat bread, or six peaches, or three apples, or two and one-half bowls of bran flakes. Prunes are, indeed, "the high fiber fruit" as the advertisements have claimed.

THERAPEUTIC BENEFITS

I recall my own experiences with green gage plums, an English variety that is green-skinned in the beginning but quickly fades to yellow and finally to bronze when fully ripened. Back in the 1970s, our family then resided in the southcentral Utah community of Manti. We had quite a row of green gage bushes on the east end of our property, next to an irrigation ditch which carried our water to several large garden plots on our one and one-half acre piece of ground.

More than once I remember going up there and eating them straight off the bushes when they started falling to the ground. They were the best physic I ever took. Within thirty minutes as a rule, the urge would come to make a necessary and rapid trip to the bathroom. I was never bothered with constipation when they came into season. Nor were the birds that feasted on them.

Back in the early 1930s the California Prune Board expended a great deal of money to exhaustively research prunes to see if they were truly laxative in nature. Two of their published studies appeared in *Proceedings of the Society for Experimental Biology and Medicine* (31:278–81, 1933–34) and *Medical Record* (February 5, 1936, pp. 117–19). They concluded that the laxative effect of prune wasn't just related to their high fiber content. They pointed out that another then unnamed substance was responsible for stimulating intestinal contractions. As proof of their hypothesis, they cited the fact that prune juice, which lacks most of the fiber of whole prunes, is still a very good laxative.

This laxative-promoting substance has since been identified as diphenylisatin. Furthermore, it helps to lower serum cholesterol levels in those suffering from mildly elevated cholesterol, according to a report in the *American Journal of Clinical Nutrition* (53:1259–65, 1991).

Gastritis. In both acute and chronic forms of this problem, the mucus lining of the stomach becomes inflamed, usually as a result of too much alcohol, spicy food, coffee, or certain drugs like aspirin. Prepared prune juice concentrate with pulp included or homemade prune juice will help provide relief. The high amount of a few mineral salts (notably potassium and magnesium) squeezes water from the colon wall and dumps it into the intestinal tract, thereby diluting these offensive foods, beverages, or drugs.

Hyperacidity. Prune juice works much like epsom salts (magnesium sulphate) does when there is an excess amount of hydrochloric acid in the gut. It squeezes water from the walls of the colon and dumps it into the G.I. tract, where it dilutes the excess acid.

METHOD OF PREPARATION

While plums and prunes, once pitted, can be juiced, I recommend purchasing the ready-made bottled or canned juices instead. They are more convenient and ready to use and can also be obtained with some of the fruit pulp in them.

POMEGRANATE JUICE

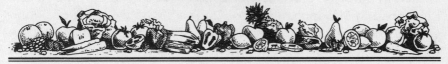

"Liquid Mouth-to-Mouth Resuscitation"

DESCRIPTION

The pomegranate is a handsome deciduous and somewhat thorny large shrub or small tree (*Punica granatum*) belonging to the family Punicaceae, native to semi-tropical Asia and naturalized in the Mediterranean region in very early times. It has long been cultivated as an ornamental and for its edible fruit.

The fruit is about the size of an average apple. A pomegranate bears numerous seeds, each within a fleshy crimson seed coating, enclosed in a tough yellowish to deep-red rind. Pomegranates are either consumed fresh or else used for grenadine syrup, in which the juice of the acid fruit pulp is the chief ingredient. Grenadine syrup, sometimes made from red currants, is a flavoring for wines, cocktails, carbonated beverages, preserves, and confectionary.

The pomegranate is now cultivated in most warm climates, to a greater extent in the Old World than in America. In North America it is grown commercially mainly from California and Arizona south into the tropics.

The fruit has long been a religious and artistic symbol. It is described in the most ancient of Asian literature. In the Old Testament, King Solomon sang of an "orchard of pomegranates." More recently, archaeologists have excavated several important unrobbed grave sites at Tel Nami, a site on the Mediterranean coast, about eight miles south of Haifa, Israel. Two foot-long, bronze scepters, decorated with incised designs and believed to have been used by officiating priests in Solomon's Temple in ancient times, were found. The heads of both scepters were carved to represent a pomegranate. A pair of gold earrings shaped like pomegranate blossoms were also located in the same grave as the scepters. Other sites at Nimrud and Khorsabad in Mesopotamia (now Iraq) showed evidence of pomegranates being symbolically used in sacrificial rites of animals. (See *Biblical Archaeology Review*, January-February 1990 and the *Israel Museum Journal* 8:7, 1989.)

NUTRITIONAL DATA

One pomegranate contains the following nutrients: 5 mg. calcium, 12 mg. phosphorus, 0.5 mg. iron, 5 mg. sodium, 399 mg. potassium, a trace of vitamin A, 6 mg. vitamin C, and 2 mg. magnesium.

THERAPEUTIC BENEFITS

Elihu Ben-David, M.D. is an Israeli physician by profession. I met him some years ago in London at an international scientific symposium devoted to medicinal plant research that we both happened to be attending at the same time. In comparing notes with each other on several different fruits and vegetables, he brought up something interesting with regard to pomegranate juice that I jotted in a small pocket notebook I had with me and have never forgotten since.

Dr. Ben-David said that in those cases where a person's heart might be too weak to sustain an individual in consciousness much longer, if such person was administered a cup of *fresh* pomegranate juice internally it would save the person from passing out altogether. He jokingly referred to pomegranate juice as "my liquid mouth-to-mouth resuscitator." Of course, he meant that it has to be given while the individual is still conscious and can swallow it, not when the person is totally unconscious and may run the risk of choking on the liquid.

Bad Breath. In parts of Iran and Iraq, squeezed pomegranate juice has been used as an effective gargle and mouthwash for halitosis due to oral thrush (yeast infection), rotting teeth, or putrid, sore throat. If it is due to fermented conditions within the gut, then a little of the juice (2 tablespoons) is diluted with some water (1 teaspoon) and swallowed for this.

Hemorrhoids. Due to its high astringency action, pomegranate juice may be applied to piles by saturating several cotton balls with the liquid before applying.

Round Worms, Pin Worms, Tapeworm. An effective treatment for intestinal worms is routinely employed in parts of Egypt and elsewhere in the Near East as well as in both Vietnams. It calls for the internal consumption of a small amount of pomegranate juice, diluted with a little water if necessary in order to make it more palatable. The rich tannin content of the juice basically stupefies the worms and causes them to be ejected from the system through the colon.

METHOD OF PREPARATION

This is one of those fruits which is better juiced than eaten raw. Because the pulp and juice cling so hard to the seeds, juicing is the easiest way to get the most from this particular fruit.

It is best to juice the entire pomegranate without peeling it. However, the liquified pulp needs to be diluted and strained through a coarse wire strainer afterwards, so that all of the seeds are removed but the juice is preserved in a pan below.

POTATO JUICE

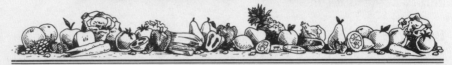

"Removing Heavy Metals from the Body"

DESCRIPTION

The potato (*Solanum tuberosum*) is the vegetable that conquered the world. Among the first Europeans to see the unimposing plant the South American Indians called *papa* were the Spanish conquistador Francisco Pizarro and his rowdy band of thugs and cutthroats. When they overran Peru in the 1530s, they were unaware of the buried treasure beneath their feet. They rode rough-shod over the papa, in hot pursuit of the Inca Atahuallpa and his fabled gold.

Introduced into Europe over the next 50 years, the incredible spud began four centuries of world conquest. The Inca Empire has long since vanished, and Spain's glory is but only a vague memory now. But King Potato keeps right on reigning. Compared to the vast benefits this versatile plant has bestowed on humanity, all the gold of Peru becomes small potatoes.

Today the potato is produced in 130 of the world's 167 independent countries. One year's crop, at consumer prices, is worth 106 billion dollars, more than the value of all the gold and silver the Spanish ever carted out of the New World. The average annual crop (291 million tons) could cover a four-lane freeway encircling the globe *six times!*

Potato plants make a growth of three feet, the branches sprawly, the stems winged, and the compound leaves having small oval leaflets with a hairy surface. The flowers are bi-sexed and borne in clusters, with a white to purple color. The seed ball, if present, is small and round. The tubers are borne on the end of short stems underground. The colors vary from white to red, and the shapes from long and slender to round.

Potatoes may be grouped into early and late varieties. There are many varieties available, and certain ones seem particularly adapted to certain localities. They may be sorted into eight or ten groups according to color and shape of the tubers and time of maturity.

A few varieties can be mentioned here. The Irish cobbler is a round, white, rather rough potato common to the heavier soils of the Atlantic Seaboard states. The early Ohio is a very early, oblong, pink-skinned potato grown in the north central states. The Burbank is a medium-late spud grown on the Pacific Coast. Baking potatoes are primarily grown west of the Mississippi River. Some have russet-colored skin, while others have clear white skins. Idaho is famous for its russet spuds that make great bakers and french fries. The Chippewa, a newer variety, is round and slightly flattened. It is rather watery and a poor keeper, but is preferred by the potato chip industry, because of its flavor and higher yield per acre.

The potato chip was invented in 1853. In Saratoga Springs, New York, short-order cook George Crum, a Native American Indian, got revenge on a customer complaining about Crum's thick fried potatoes. He defiantly prepared a batch of superthin slices and deep fried them. The rest, as they say, is history. French fries were introduced to America when Thomas Jefferson served them in the White House. The man who pioneered our modern use of the frozen french fry, though, was Idaho's own potato king, the late J.R. "Jack" Simplot.

Years ago when I lived and worked in Idaho Falls, Idaho, from 1968–1970, I met Mr. Simplot one time at the Westbank Restaurant where I then worked as a chef. I remember him telling me, "Son, I never met a potato I didn't like!"

NUTRITIONAL DATA

The potato is so nutritious that a man in Scandinavia lived healthily for 300 days on only spuds dressed with a tad of margarine. It takes seven pounds of spuds, about 23, to total 2,500 calories, the estimated adult daily requirement; so eating a spud without rich toppings is no more fattening than eating a pear—the potato itself is 99.9 percent fat free.

An acre of potatoes yields almost as much food as two acres of grain, and when the water that composes about 80% of potatoes is squeezed out, they provide annually more edible dry matter than the combined worldwide consumption of fish and meat.

Potatoes are especially high in mineral content with the heaviest concentrations being in the skins. The science journal *Acta Agriculturae Scandinavica* (Supplement 22, 1980) reported that "the concentrations are generally at their highest in raw unpeeled potato and at their lowest in potato peeled before cooking. The following nutritional data obtained from this same journal is for one raw, unpeeled potato: 27.3 mg. potassium, 0.258 mg. calcium, 1.13 mg. magnesium, 2.93 mg. phosphorus, 1.63 mg. sulphur, 28.3 mg. iron, 3.37 mg. copper, 12.7 mg. manganese, 20 mg. zinc, 0.2 mg. molybdenum, 0.02 mg. cobalt, 0.14 mg. nickel, 0.04 mg. chromium, 0.8 mg. fluorine, 0.01 mg. selenium, 10 mg. silicon, 15.3 mg. rubidium, 15 mg. aluminum, 7.1 mg. boron, 2 mg. bromine, 0.004 mg. mercury, 0.05 mg. arsenic, 0.07 mg. cadmium, and 0.110 mg. lead. Some of these minerals which are considered to be toxic in large amounts, such as aluminum, arsenic, mercury and lead, are essential to the body in very minute quantities and appeared in the potatoes analyzed for this study because of the rich, uncontaminated soils in which they were grown.

THERAPEUTIC BENEFITS

Science is one of a large number of scientific journals which I regularly subscribe to and routinely read in the search for new information that will enable me to help others more. In one back issue almost a decade ago (230:603; 674–76, Nov. 8, 1985), I read about certain plants containing simple peptides called phytochelatins, that bind heavy metals and thus participate in metal detoxification.

Scientists made cultures of cells from several different plant species. Among them were dill, eggplant, potato, bedstraw, marshmallow, and barberry. Toxic heavy metals such as cadmium, copper, mercury, lead, and zinc were then added to these various cell cultures. "More than 90 percent of the cadmium put into cultures became complexed with phytochelatins," the journal noted. When such heavy metals are complexed with three simple sulphur amino acids, they become harmless and are detoxified out of the body if they occur in too great an abundance.

Based on this and corresponding research published elsewhere since then, I have always recommended potato juice for heavy metal toxicity. My own experience with it has been that it is one of the very best agents for pulling those metallic elements out of body tissue, which can accumulate there over a lengthy period of time and can lead to severe health problems later on.

Blackheads, Boils, Cysts, Carbuncles. The heavy starch content of potato juice and the pulp makes a wonderful drawing agent to pull purulent matter right out of the system. First, the particular eruption needs to be carefully lanced with a sewing needle that has been sterilized over a flame for a minute. Then, a small square section of muslin, cotton, or flannel cloth (about the size of a folded handkerchief) is thoroughly soaked in potato juice and pulp. It is then applied directly to the skin and covered by another piece of clean, white cloth (preferably folded once). This cataplasm is kept in place for awhile until it dries out; then another is applied. Following this treatment, the surface of the skin is washed and then disinfected with some hydrogen peroxide. Several applications may be necessary in order to pull out as much poison as possible.

Bedsores, Diabetic Leg Ulcers, Wounds. The same aforementioned routine is prescribed here, except that the intended area of treatment doesn't need to be lanced. This also works well on genital herpes sores. Afterwards, the site should be treated with some vinegar or white hazel to not only disinfect but also help to close up the sore or wound.

Gallstones. When I was a very young boy, for some strange reason I came down with a case of severe gallstones. My father consulted a naturopathic doctor, who recommended the same thing which his mother, Barbara Liebhardt Heinerman, had used years before in the Old Country (Temesvár, Romania). This was the internal administration of raw potato juice, as well as cooked potato peeling broth. I was given half cupfuls of both at different intervals throughout the day for nearly a week. All of the gallstones were discharged through my colon and I recovered nicely. But oh, yecch! How I wish my father had flavored that potato juice and peeling broth a little!

METHOD OF PREPARATION

When juicing any potato, there is one very important thing to keep in mind: Under no circumstances should you peel it. You may wash it with soap and water if you like, even lightly scrub it with a wire vegetable brush. But *don't* ever peel it, because that's where all of the mineral nourishment that will flush poisons out of your system lies.

If using a Vita-Mix, I suggest that you cut the spud into small quarter sections for easier juicing with a little water added while doing so. If using some other type of juicing machine, you only need to cut the spud lengthwise in half.

PUMPKIN JUICE

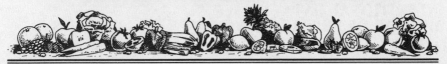

"Boost Your Health with Vitamin A"

DESCRIPTION

Pumpkins fall into two basic groups: one (*Cucurbita pepo*), includes the common summer and autumn pumpkins and the bush pumpkins, and the other (*Cucurbita moschata*), embraces the winter crookneck pumpkins. That pumpkins are closely related to their cousins the squashes (*Cucurbita maxima*) is well illustrated by the fact that many pumpkins, such as the pattypan and summer squash, are commonly called squashes.

The difference in foliage and fruit characters of the two species of pumpkins as contrasted with the squashes should be clearly noted. Pumpkins have coarse, harsh, large, deeply lobed or entire leaves on bushy or trailing vines. The flowers are always large and funnel-shaped, with orange-yellow petals. The fruits vary tremendously in size, shape, and color. The seeds are flat and oblong, with a gentle taper toward either end. Pumpkins are native to Central and South America, as is the squash.

Pumpkin varieties include: the Connecticut field, which is a large, orange pumpkin with slight ribbing, weighing around 50 pounds, from which many Halloween jack-o-lanterns are carved; the sugar pumpkin which is golden-yellow or brownish-yellow and flattened, weighs just four to five pounds, but makes great juice or pie filling; crookneck squash which is either white or yellow in color and has a warted skin when ripe; and zucchini bush pumpkin which is synonymous with zucchini squash (see the very last juice entry in this book).

NUTRITIONAL DATA

One pound of canned pumpkin pulp contains the following nutrients: 113 mg. calcium, 118 mg. phosphorus, 1.8 mg. iron, 9 mg. sodium, 1,089 mg. potassium, 29,030 I.U. vitamin A, 2.7 mg. niacin, 23 mg. vitamin C, and 66 mg. magnesium.

THERAPEUTIC BENEFITS

During the weekend of August 13-15, 1982, I gave an extensive workshop at the Natural Health Ranch in Tunnel Hill, Georgia. It was widely promoted, including an interview with me by reporter George W. Brown from the *Chattanooga News-Free Press.*

Mr. Sam Waters read about it in this newspaper and came all the way from Sweetwater, Tennessee to hear my concluding lecture on Sunday. I mentioned how boiled pumpkin juice had been used by some Hopi and Zuni Indian folk healers in Arizona to treat various cases of leukemia with modest success. He wondered aloud if the *raw* juice might not work even better in such instances. My reply was that I couldn't see how it would hurt to at least try it.

Waters, who suffered from leukemia in the early stages, went back home, purchased a juicer (he later told me) and proceeded to make himself fresh pumpkin and crookneck squash juices that he drank faithfully every day. About five months later, he dropped me a short note to say that his "improved Indian remedy" (as he liked to call it) had worked "health miracles" and totally "cured me of my leukemia."

A few years later as the AIDS epidemic spread and gained more notoriety with the media, I was asked to do a series of workshops in West Los Angeles with Dr. Laurence Badgley, a holistic physician from Foster City (just below San Francisco) who specialized in exclusively treating members of the gay community who suffered from this terrible disease. I was introduced to one young man, whom

I'll call Joe to preserve his real identity, who had Kaposi sarcoma (one of the usual symptoms of AIDS).

Dr. Badgley had already put him on a pretty strenuous and restricted dietary and nutritional program. Joe was responding to some extent, but not as much as Dr. Badgley had hoped he would. Further tests showed that Joe's liver still wasn't quite functioning like it should, even with all that he was then doing right. Dr. Badgley conferred with me on the matter, and I advised him to have Joe start drinking two cups of pumpkin juice every day with meals, because, I said, "this will give your patient a whopping amount of beta-carotene which his system can rapidly assimilate and, in turn, give his undernourished liver a badly needed boost." This was done according to my instructions and soon a noticeable improvement in Joe's progress was made. Today, as of this writing in late 1993, Joe is still alive and takes pride in being a long-term survivor of AIDS. Certainly, pumpkin juice alone didn't do it, but the entire program Dr. Badgley put him on was what has worked for him in his amazing battle with a disease that is most often terminal.

Vitamin A Deficiency.   Pumpkin juice is literally "loaded to the gills" with an abundance of vitamin A. In fact, I challenge you to find another vegetable (except maybe for carrots) with an equivalent amount of beta-carotene. You can never overdose on this form of vitamin A, except that your skin might turn slightly yellow-orange in the process. In cases of allergies, skin problems, vision disorders, blood sugar imbalances, infections, joint swelling, lung problems, elevated cholesterol and triglyceride levels, and liver disturbances, this is the juice to be drinking every day. If it tastes a little odd, then dilute it with some carrot or mixed chlorophyll juice to improve the flavor.

METHOD OF PREPARATION

Before portions of a pumpkin can be juiced, they need to be peeled of their outer hard shell and the seeds removed. A mastication juice machine such as the Champion is best for something like this, where the raw material you're working with is pretty tough and hard. Be advised that the taste will be somewhat strange and different to your palate. It may, therefore, be necessary to dilute the pumpkin juice with a little carrot juice or liquid chlorophyll to flavor it up a bit. I recommend *no more* than two cups per day on account of the very high vitamin A content present.

QUINCE JUICE

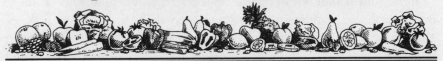

"Antidote for Montezuma's Revenge"

DESCRIPTION

The common quince (*Cydonia oblonga*) is a spineless tree with edible fruits cultivated from ancient times in the Orient and in the Mediterranean area, where it was naturalized. Its pome fruit is similar to that of the related apple and pear but is very astringent, and hence it is used chiefly cooked in preserves; marmalade was first made from quince some food historians say.

As a commercial fruit tree, the quince is cultivated more widely in the temperate zone of Europe than in the United States, where it is grown mainly in California and New York. It is often used as a rootstock for dwarf fruit trees, especially the pear. The flowering quinces are cultivated as ornamental shrubs for their profuse, usually thorny branches and attractive scarlet, pink, or white flowers. The fruit is too small and hard to be of much commercial value except for local use.

NUTRITIONAL DATA

One ripe quince contains the following nutrients: 10 mg. calcium, 16 mg. phosphorus, 0.64 mg. iron, 4 mg. sodium, 181 mg. potassium, 37 I.U. vitamin A, 13.8 mg. vitamin C, and 7 mg. magnesium.

THERAPEUTIC BENEFITS

I have been to most of the countries on the Pacific Rim for research, lecturing, and consulting work. From May 19–21, 1986 I was in Taipei Taiwan attending The Joint Conference of The Second World Congress of Chinese Medicine and Pharmacy. This was a huge international symposium sponsored by the Dept. of Health of Taiwan and the China Medical College in Taipei. Over one thousand delegates were in attendance. Along with many others I presented an important scientific paper on an aspect of my work with botanical medicine.

During this historic weekend event, I had the good fortune of meeting other colleagues, who like myself, were doing research on fruits, vegetables, herbs, and medicinal mushrooms. Among them was Hsin Sheng Tsay, who shared with me some remarkable things he had been doing with quince fruit.

Tsay found that the juice of the quince was wonderful for stopping even the worst kinds of diarrhea. He presented several case studies involving three Oriental women and two men, for whom nothing else had worked except this particular fruit juice. Admittedly, the juice is somewhat sour due to its astringency, but it is this very quality that makes it such a marvelous anti-diarrheal.

The proverbial "loose bowels" that American tourists often experience while visiting Mexico, is no stranger to the Orient. In fact, "Montezuma's revenge" exists in many Third World countries where the sanitary conditions of the food and water might be in question. His research has shown that for those suffering from this embarrassing and fatiguing problem in the Middle East, Nepal, Pakistan, India, mainland China, Taiwan, Japan, Thailand, Vietnam, and similar places, quince fruit is readily available as an effective natural food-medicine to promptly cure it.

Cholera. This is an acute epidemic infectious disease caused by *Vibrio cholerae*, now occurring primarily in Asia. One major symptom is a profuse watery diarrhea. Some Oriental herbalists and alternative-minded doctors prescribe quince juice for their patients suffering from cholera. This seems to prevent the dangers inherent with the onset of dehydration by quickly and effectively stopping the diarrhea.

Dysentery (Amebic). This is a condition of prolonged diarrhea resulting from ulcerative inflammation of the colon, caused chiefly by infection with *Entamoeba histolytica.* Quince juice can halt the diarrhea and stop the infection because of its strong astringent properties.

Lice. Any of three vegetable juices noted for their potent astringency properties, is good to wash the scalp or body with in order to get rid of lice. These would be persimmon, pomegranate, and quince juices.

METHOD OF PREPARATION

The green fruit is the best to juice for quickly solving diarrhea. Only a little bit needs to be taken internally for this, probably half a cup which is what Dr. Tsay employed most often. In some instances, however, he would have to administer double this amount, always on an empty stomach. The astringency factor is at its highest state while the fruit is still unripe. This declines as the fruit matures.

Here is an "all-purpose" remedy made from quince juice that is popular in some parts of the Orient. Put the following measured ingredients into a stainless steel pot, ceramic jug, or small oak flask and soak for $1\frac{1}{2}$ months, then strain and bottle: $1\frac{1}{4}$ quarts quince juice, 1 cup crushed litchi seeds (also spelled leechee, lichee, and lychee), 1 tbsp. crushed bitter almond, pinches of mace, cinnamon, and ginger, two cups of fine brandy, and $\frac{1}{4}$ tsp. powdered cloves.

RADISH JUICE

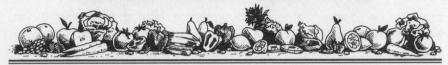

"Nutrition for the Thyroid"

DESCRIPTION

The garden radish (*Raphanus sativus*) is one of the easiest vegetables to grow and is probably in more gardens than any other vegetable. It is a native of Asia and has been in cultivation for many centuries, having been highly prized by ancient Egyptian pharaohs and the early Greeks. In Jürgen Thorwald's book *Science and Secrets of Early Medicine* (New York: Harcourt, Brace & World, Inc., 1962; p. 92) is mentioned a report given by the ancient Greek historian Herodotus in the 5th century B.C. concerning the pyramid builders: "There is an inscription in Egyptian characters on the pyramid which records the quantity of radishes, onions, and garlic consumed by the labourers who constructed it; and I perfectly well remember that the interpreter who read the writing to me said that the money thus expended was 1600 talents of silver [equivalent to about $4 million today]."

During the days of minimum sunlight, the radish plant produces a rosette of leaves and a thick, very tender taproot of various dimensions and colors, and as the days become longer, it sends out a tall branching seedstalk with small purplish white flowers. Radish seed sown in late summer produces good radishes which do not make a seedstalk until the following spring. (See also Horseradish Juice.)

Radishes come in assorted colors, shapes, and sizes. The most common ones are of the small, red, globe-shaped variety and are marketed either in bunches with their green tops attached or in cellophane bags (usually six ounces) without the greens. The bunched radishes are harvested and bunched by hand, then packed with crushed ice and rushed to market. They are fairly perishable and must be sold within a few days of picking or the tender green tops start to break down. If those tops are withered, and especially if they have started to turn yellow, it's a dead giveaway that the radishes aren't fresh. In some areas, these tops, provided they are fresh and green, are highly prized as a salad green.

For juicing purposes, it is best to use bunched radishes that include these green leafy tops.

There are also some radishes that are pure white in color. One of these is rather large and looks like a huge albino carrot. It is an unusual radish of Oriental origin and is called a daikon radish. Until recently it could only be found in Oriental food stores but now are available in most large supermarkets.

Then there are black radishes, which look like huge, ebony-colored beets in size. But beneath their unattractive exterior lies a pure white flesh that is crisp in texture and has a sharp zesty flavor. They have a long shelf life and, if stored in a cool area, stay firm and

Radishes

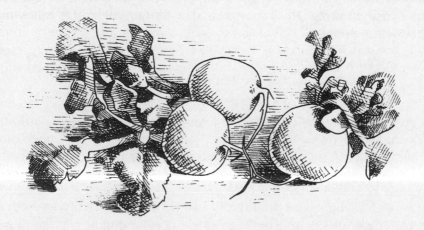

fresh for months on end. Black radishes are widely used in Eastern Europe. In the U.S. they are primarily sold in markets that serve large ethnic Russian and Polish clientele.

NUTRITIONAL DATA

Ten large red radishes (minus their tops) yield the following nutrients: 24 mg. calcium, 25 mg. phosphorus, 0.8 mg. iron, 15 mg. sodium, 261 mg. potassium, 10 I.U. vitamin A, 21 mg. vitamin C, 4 mg. magnesium, 2 mg. selenium, and 0.13 mg. zinc.

THERAPEUTIC BENEFITS

The thyroid is a butterfly-shaped gland located at the base of the neck, just below the larynx and in front of the windpipe (trachea). Its two lobes straddle the latter and are connected by a thin strip of tissue. The thyroid manufactures an important hormone called thyroxine (or T_4). This hormone's role is to stimulate or regulate almost all of the body's metabolic processes and many of its other functions.

The late Henry G. Bieler, M.D. was more specific about the importance of the thyroid gland in his book *Food is Your Best Medicine* (New York: Random House, 1966; pp. 43;72). He plainly stated that a healthy thyroid was imperative to successful weight loss in obese subjects. He also noted that T_4 facilitated the following bodily functions:

- cell production
- oxidation in all of the body tissues
- repair of damaged/diseased body tissues
- sugar liberation from the liver to the blood stream
- the heart beat
- brain and special sense activity
- normal cell growth

In fact, he called the thyroid gland, "nature's own pace setter" which determined whether the body's cellular engines "poke along or race dangerously fast."

Black radishes have been used by some doctors in the old Soviet Union as accepted medical treatment for hypothyroidism and hyperthyroidism. With the former, the thyroid is deficient in producing adequate amounts of thyroxine; whereas with the latter (also known as Graves' disease), too much is being produced. During my historic 1979 mid-summer trip to the old Soviet Union, by invitation of the Soviet Academy of Sciences, I had a chance to interview several medical experts considered very proficient in the uses of vegetable and herbal materia medica for treating diseases.

What they told me about the effects of radishes (both red and black) on the thyroid, was nothing short of amazing! Raphanin, the main sulphur component in radishes, is chiefly responsible for keeping the production of thyroxine and calcitonin (a peptide hormone) in normal balance. With enough raphanin circulating in the blood plasma through a steady diet of radishes or radish juice, the thyroid won't under- or over-produce these two hormones. Wherever there has been a thyroid problem somewhere brought to my attention, I've always thought back on this information I learned from my trip to the former U.S.S.R., and, as a consequence, have routinely recommended a few radishes in the diet every day or else a *very small* amount of radish juice (often mixed in with another vegetable juice such as carrot, tomato, celery or zucchini). Sometimes, for good measure, I will even suggest adding a little powdered or granulated kelp (about one half teaspoonful) for good measure. (Kelp is a seaweed obtained from health food stores and is rich in iodine and other trace elements which benefit the thyroid gland a lot.)

Constipation. Some German doctors have routinely used small amounts of fresh radish juice to gently stimulate peristalsis so that bowel evacuation can be promoted. It is usually diluted with a little cabbage, celery, parsley, or watercress juice.

Fatty Liver Disease. This is a buildup of fat deposits in the liver, causing it to become enlarged. Diabetes, Reye's syndrome, obesity, chemical toxins, and high fat intake are responsible for this condition. The sulphur amino acids in radish juice help to break up the fat deposits in the liver. The juice should be made fresh every day, not stored for any length of time in the refrigerator. Also, radish juice must be diluted with a secondary vegetable juice (e.g., carrot, chlorophyll, tomato).

Gallbladder Inflammation.   The late German author, Rudolf Fritz Weiss, M.D., stated in the 6th edition of his *Lehrbuch der Phytothera-pie* (Stuttgart: Hippokrates Verlag GmbH, 1985; p. 94) that "radish juice may be initiated at the sub-acute stage of cholecystitis ..." However, the radish juice still needs to be diluted with a secondary vegetable juice so as to make it more acceptable to the digestive tract.

METHOD OF PREPARATION

When juicing radishes, it is best to use those which are bunched or gathered fresh and sold while still quite fresh with their green tops intact. These make the best kind of radish juice and also contains the highest amount of minerals. The late Norman Walker, who died at an age somewhere over 100, cautioned in his book, *Fresh Vegetable and Fruit Juices* (Prescott, AZ: Norwalk Press, 1986; p. 58) that radish juice "should never be taken alone, as it is too strong in its reaction if taken by itself. Walker advised that it be combined with something like carrot juice to make it more agreeable to the system.

   If using a juicer such as a Vita-Mix, you may want to chop the radishes into tiny pieces so they juice easier; but if you have another type of juicer this won't be necessary to do.

RHUBARB JUICE

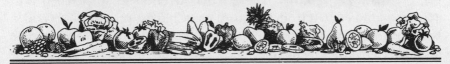

"The Dentist's Friend"

DESCRIPTION

The common rhubarb (*Rheum rhaponticum*) used for making pies is a native of Southern Siberia. It is a perennial, herbaceous plant which is grown for its fleshy petioles, commonly referred to as stalks. The leaves are very large and somewhat heart-shaped and the petioles are two to six feet tall, depending on where the plant is grown. The leafstalks are harvested in the summer, before the seedstalk is sent up. The flowers are born on a cluster on the tall stem and are greenish white in color. The crown of the plant is a rhizome with many-branched, large, fleshy roots.

Rhubarb was rarely recognized as a food until about three centuries ago. Just as the tomato is a fruit but is referred to as a vegetable, the rhubarb is a vegetable but is thought of as a fruit, especially when associated with pies and sauces. Confusion may also come from the fact that it is especially good when cooked with strawberries, a type of fruit.

There are two basic types of rhubarb: outdoor and hothouse. Outdoor rhubarb comes in season in spring and lasts until fall. The stalks are often more green than red and have large, floppy, green leaves. It is quite coarse in texture and often springy. It is also very tart and requires a lot of sugar. The hothouse variety, which is produced in California, Oregon, and Michigan arrives in January and finishes up in June. It is either cherry-red or blushing-pink. Some hothouse rhubarb have bright yellow leaves and are particularly attractive. It is not as stringy as outdoor rhubarb, has a milder flavor, and requires less sugar. Rhubarb leaves, however, should not be consumed.

Some American herb companies used a medicinal rhubarb from China (*Rheum officinale*). There it has been used since 2000 B.C. The best kind comes from the northern Chinese province of Gansu, which borders the Mongolian People's Republic. The soil and climate are just right for giving this medicinal rhubarb its reddish-yellow color, firm texture, deep yellow tinge, and smooth, bitter-sharp flavor. I have never seen this variety juiced, only used in powder, pill or capsule forms.

NUTRITIONAL DATA

One cup of chopped rhubarb contains the following nutrients: 105 mg. calcium, 17 mg. phosphorus, 0.27 mg. iron, 5 mg. sodium, 351 mg. potassium, 122 I.U. vitamin A, 8.7 mg. folic acid, 9.8 mg. vitamin C, and 14 mg. magnesium.

THERAPEUTIC BENEFITS

An Amish lady by the name of Mrs. Byler—I never got her first name—wrote to me some time ago from Smicksburg, Pennsylvania. Her family was bothered with various dental problems, which she listed for me in her letter, and she wanted to know what could be done about them. Her husband had rather bad tooth discoloration due to the nicotine from the cigars he smoked and the tobacco he chewed. She suffered from a continual buildup of dental plaque and tartar. Her several children had bouts with different types of teeth and gum disease (caries, gingivitis, and pyorrhea). Her little five-year-old also had a bad case of thrush on his tongue (a form of candidiasis or yeast infection). She wanted to know what could be done for all of these problems.

Ordinarily, I would have recommended four or five different things to cover all they had. But, fortunately, I was familiar with a relatively new product from Pines International of Lawrence, Kansas that is still a pretty well kept secret in most of the health food industry.

Owner Ron Seibold was given a start of a particular variety of rhubarb from a family in Concordia, Kansas a few years ago, who had grown it for four generations themselves. Their pioneer ancestors brought it from the same state in which Mrs. Byler lived in the mid-19th century.

Ron's grower harvests this special rhurbarb only once a year. The juice is quickly extracted from the fleshy stalks and spray dried with arrowroot. Pine's rhubarb juice power has a sweet-tart flavor about it much like homemade lemonade does but without the added sugar. Knowing that rhubarb juice is quite "user friendly" when it comes to oral problems and that Amish don't have electricity for kitchen equipment like a juice machine, I sent her a bottle of Pines' new product with simple instructions on how to use it.

I advised her to have everyone in the family brush their teeth, gums and tongues every day with this juice powder. They were to wet their toothbrushes first, before dipping them into some of this powder. They were to do this twice or three times daily without fail for six weeks and then to report back the results to me.

Before two months had ended, she wrote back to say that her husband's teeth were whiter, that her plaque was gone although some tartar buildup still remained, that her children's dental health had vastly improved, and that the thrush had entirely cleared up in the mouth of her youngest child. She exclaimed, "Rhubarb is trewly [sic] the dentist's best friend."

The reader should understand that *raw* rhubarb juice contains oxalic acid which isn't good for the body when swallowed too frequently. William H. Lee, author of *The Book of Raw Fruit and Vegetable Juices and Drinks* (New Canaan: Keats Publishing, Inc., 1982; p. 64) warned: "Rhubarb is not a friend to man; I was tempted to leave it out of [my] book altogether..." So use it very judiciously. But, as I said before, the Pines' juice product is very "user friendly" for oral problems and can be used this way without any concern.

Rhubarb juice can be applied as a poultice or wash externally or taken in very small amounts internally for these few problems:

bedsores	intestinal gas
constipation	intestinal parasites
gangrene	leg ulcers
hemorrhaging	wounds

Those suffering from kidney stones should not use rhubarb juice!

Bed Sores, Diabetic Leg Ulcers, Wounds.   Make a paste out of ½ teaspoon Pines' rhubarb juice powder and ¼ teaspoon honey. Apply to sores, skin ulcers and wounds. This will accelerate healing.

Diarrhea.   One tablespoon of Pine's rhubarb juice powder mixed in one glass (8 fl. oz.) of water should remedy mild diarrhea *not* caused by bacterial infections.

METHOD OF PREPARATION

Rhubarb petioles can still be juiced if one so desires. Because they are so tough and fibrous, a machine like a Champion juicer would make juicing much easier over other models. However, Pines' rhubarb juice powder is highly recommended as an efficient and convenient substitute for the petioles. (See Appendix Four for more information.)

SPINACH JUICE

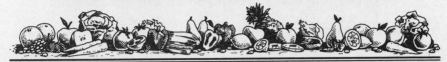

"Worried About Wrinkles? Try this Elixir"

DESCRIPTION

Spinach (*Spinacia oleracea*) has always been the favorite food of the cartoon screen character, Popeye the Sailor Man. Whenever in trouble and at his wit's end, he would reach inside his uniform and pull out a can of spinach, pop it open somehow, and in one mighty gulp swallow the entire contents. A moment later his muscles would bulge in every direction and he would become temporarily transformed into a sort of superman, using his incredible found strength to save himself and others from harm's way and to dispense whatever justice was necessary to evil wrongdoers such as his hulking nemesis named Brutus.

What Max Fleischman, the creator of Popeye, Olive Oyl, Wimpy, and the other cartoon characters, failed to tell the millions of children who grew up watching them on television every Saturday morning, was that spinach doesn't taste that great!

It is a fleshy-leafed annual that forms a heavy rosette of broad, crinkly, tender leaves, very high in vitamin and mineral contents. During hot weather, spinach sends up a flowering stalk with long pointed leaves which bear inconspicuos male or female flowers. Spinach originally came from Asia and eastern Europe, but is now grown in just about every corner of the globe.

There are many varieties of spinach, but they can be broken down into three groups: the savoy, which has crinkly leaves, the semi-savoy, which has leaves that aren't as crinkly; and the flat leaf. All three types are crisp and dark green when fresh and limp and yellow when aged.

NUTRITIONAL DATA

One cup of finely chopped spinach is a nutritional powerhouse for these important minerals and vitamins: 51 mg. calcium, 28 mg. phosphorus, 1.7 mg. iron, 39 mg. sodium, 259 mg. potassium, 4,460 I.U. vitamin A, 28 mg. vitamin C, 3.5 mg. biotin, 1.25 mg. vitamin E, 44 mg. magnesium, 0.42 mg. manganese, and 0.5 mg. zinc.

THERAPEUTIC BENEFITS

Fran R. is a midwife who lives just outside of Douglas, Georgia. Her practice is based on a lifetime of experience instead of a few years cramming the books at some college for a degree that would earn her a medical license for what she does. "I deliver babies just fine but I don't have me a piece of paper that says I can do it l-e-g-a-l," she points out, giving the last word deliberate emphasis. That's why she asked that I use her nickname and an abbreviation instead of her real name.

In the foods and herbs which she has recommended to newly pregnant moms to help them minimize the risks attached to childbirth, she discovered that spinach and spinach juice helped to reduce the incidence of birth defects and miscarriages dramatically. Because Fran often travels great distances to render her services to mothers in need, she has seen more than her share of problem births. "Miscarriages are the hardest thing for a mother to handle," she told me. "It's like losing the life you never got to know, never got a chance to get close to. Like losing a part of yourself, in fact."

"Don't ask me how it works," she shrugs. "I dunno. All I know is that the spinach works. Those who take the spinach regularly have more normal births, less problems you know. In cases where they can't always get the spinach, I give them the canned spinach juice to drink. I just knows it works. You're the big man with the fancy degree and title. *You* tell me how it works." I offer the same helpless shrug in reply to her statement.

But Fran did tell me that three to four "good helpings" of steamed or cooked spinach greens a week (including the water it's cooked in) or 3 glasses of canned spinach juice a week with meals, "is what seems to do the trick in preventing them 'birth accidents,'" she states with an authoritative air about her.

Anemia.   Spinach juice has adequate levels of iron which can help alleviate some of the problems associated with anemia.

Fatigue.   Iron depletion in women is greater than in men because of their monthly periods. Fatigue is, therefore, more common with them. Spinach juice diluted with an equal amount of carrot or tomato will provide sufficient iron to boost women's energy levels.

Wrinkles.   Take several cotton balls and bunch them together. Then soak them in some spinach juice and rub in a circular motion around the corners of the eyes, across the forehead, around the corners of the mouth, and down the chin. Do this for five minutes upon getting up in the morning and before retiring at night. Afterwards, rinse the face with cold water and then rub in some persimmon or pomegranate juice using the same technique. This procedure will help to tighten the skin and get rid of about 40-60% of existing wrinkles.

METHOD OF PREPARATION

Wash some fresh spinach leaves under running water to thoroughly clean them. If using a Vita-Mix, set the first control on variable low and the second knob on the number 2 or 3 position. It may be a good idea to add half a cup of water to dilute the thickness of the juice. Because spinach juice contains a small amount of oxalic acid, it may be good to mix it with a secondary vegetable juice, such as carrot, tomato, Wakunaga's Kyo-Green, or Pines' powdered beet concentrate (see Appendix 3).

STRING BEAN JUICE

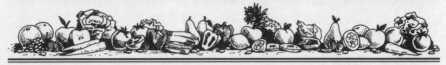

"Health Marvel for Diabetes and Hypoglycemia"

DESCRIPTION

The common bean (*Phaseolus* species) embraces the wide variety of garden beans, known as snap beans, string beans, green beans, or wax beans; the field beans, which are shelled and dried and include the red kidney beans and the small navy beans; and the Spanish frijoles as well as the French haricots.

The bean was found in cultivation by the original Native American tribes when the Western Hemisphere was first discovered by Spanish and Portuguese explorers several centuries ago. It was they and the Jesuit missionaries who accompanied them to the New World, that caused the bean to be taken to other parts of the globe. It is one of our most popular vegetables, upwards of 500 varieties being in cultivation.

It is a legume, able to obtain its nitrogen from the air, and is therefore often used as a rotation crop for soil-improvement, the vines being plowed under to fertilize the succeeding crop. The flowers are white, pink, yellow, or red. The plants range in habit of growth from low and bushy to tall and climbing, and are accordingly classified as either "bush" or "pole" varieties.

Garden beans (*Phaseolus vulgata*) are the snap, string, green, or wax beans mentioned earlier that are commonly grown in

252

household gardens for their immature edible pods. They come in either the bush or pole varieties, although the former are by far the most popular, because they are grown with so little effort.

Identifying tender green or wax beans of top quality is a snap. If they don't snap, don't buy them. Professional produce buyers determine the quality of the bean by the way it feels. A young, tender bean will have a pliable velvety feel. Only buy beans that feel fresh and look colorful. Avoid those that look or feel coarse and dried out or are discolored.

NUTRITIONAL DATA

One cup of fresh-picked string beans yields the following important nutrients: 41 mg. calcium, 42 mg. phosphorus, 1.14 mg. iron, 6 mg. sodium, 230 mg. potassium, 735 I.U. vitamin A, 40 mg. folic acid, 17.9 mg. vitamin C, and 27 mg. magnesium.

THERAPEUTIC BENEFITS

I knew the late Paavo Airola, N.D., Ph.D. He was born in Finland and educated in naturopathic medicine in England and Sweden. He spent a decade of his life carefully studying biological medicine, nutrition and what was then considered to be unorthodox treatments for illness in famous European clinics and health spas. Dr. Airola eventually came to America where he developed a large following through his dozen or so books, numerous public speaking appearances, and thriving clinical practices.

He could be arrogant, imperialistic, and wholly unaccommodating to the lay person, but cordial, practical, and almost respectful with his peers. He died a few years ago in midday on a busy sidewalk in Phoenix, Arizona of a ruptured aneurysm.

Paavo *knew* his stuff, though, and for that he earned my admiration. He was not only a student of nature, but also an *observer* of the same as well.

I remember sometime in the early 1980s meeting him at a National Health Federation Convention in Phoenix, where we both shared the speaking platform but at different hours. In a private discussion with him on blood sugar problems, I remember to this day him telling me quite pointedly with a raised pinky for emphasis: "There is *nothing*, I mean *nothing* better for diabetes or hypoglycemia than string bean juice. I make my patients take it faithfully, one cup morning, late morning, afternoon, mid-afternoon, and in the evening with each of their *five* small meals. People with blood sugar imbalances should *not* be eating three big meals a day, but instead spread them over an extended period and consume five smaller meals. Other vegetable juices are good for them to take, but I *always* emphasize this juice *first*! Why? Because of all the fruits and vegetables I know of, string bean juice alone resuscitates the pancreas, spleen and liver better than anything else I've prescribed. *No* diabetic or hypoglycemic should ever be without it!"

Paavo sincerely believed and *knew* from tests which he had conducted as a biologist on some of his patients, that string bean juice stimulated the islets of Langerhans which are scattered across the interstitial tissue of the pancreas. Therefore, stringbean juice regularly, five small meals per day, and *"lots of exercise"* were his three principal prescriptions for every diabetic and hypoglycemic he met and successfully treated.

Alcoholism.   The liver is always adversely affected with the over-consumption of alcohol. Equal parts of fresh string bean and tomato juice (fresh, canned or bottled) will help to revive this organ.

Drug Addiction.   The liver is damaged whenever illicit or legal drugs are used in excess. One third parts string bean juice, carrot juice (fresh or canned), and Kyo-Green from Wakunaga will assist this organ in recuperating from this type of abuse.

Uremic Poisoning.   String bean juice, when mixed with another vegetable drink of some type, will help to neutralize an excess of urea and other nitrogenous waste matter showing up in the blood stream.

METHOD OF PREPARATION

One definite advantage in juicing string beans is that you don't have
to snip off the stems. After washing them in a colander under running
water, just throw in your Vita-Mix with a little added water or run
through any other juice machine you may have on hand. Don't be
afraid to use the stem, peel, leaves, and seeds. *Everything* is good
with string beans. I suggest mixing half a glass with one quarter
carrot, Pines' beet powder concentrate, or Wakunaga's Kyo-Green.
Any of those three will make one therapeutic glass of juice, bar none!

TOMATO JUICE

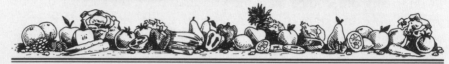

"Bugle Call for Waking Up the Liver"

DESCRIPTION

Perhaps the most popular and widely grown vegetable is the garden tomato (*Lycopersicon esculentum*). It is grown in most parts of the world and a tremendous quantity is canned for worldwide distribution. It is a native of tropical America and the fruit, formerly referred to as the gold apple and love apple, was once considered poisonous. The plants are succulent annuals, much-branched, with compound leaves having many leaflets, and small, perfect, yellow-petaled flowers produced in clusters of from three to a dozen or more in long racemes. The fruits may be as small as a currant or as large as a small pumpkin, and the shapes include the berry, pear, plum, heart, apple, and the large flat fruits that weigh over two pounds. The colors include the white, yellow, pink, and red varieties.

There has always been some dispute as to whether the tomato is a fruit or a vegetable. Since it is technically a berry it is botanically classified as a fruit. However, in the marketplace it is always classified as a vegetable by the consumer, and the customer is always right. So for practical purposes here we'll settle for it being a vegetable, though it really isn't.

Vine-ripened and force-ripened tomatoes both look alike, but there are worlds of difference in their respective tastes. The former

256

"smell" slightly alkaline if you hold one up close to your nose and sniff the top stem end where it had clung to the vine before being picked. Cut one open and you can immediately detect the pleasant mineral flavor which needs no further salting to be enjoyed. On the other hand, supermarket tomatoes are picked while still grass-green. After which they're washed, graded, and packed by machine, then eventually exposed to warmth and gassed with ethylene oxide; the combination of the two force-ripens all the way from pink to a rosy-red. They taste like sawdust and often are too hard to be juicy like the vine-ripened ones get.

Growers prefer force-ripened because it means a lot more cash for their crops. Labor costs are just a fraction of those needed to produce vine-ripened tomatoes. There is also a far greater yield per acre because there is less chance of damage in the field from rain, wind, or hail, and there is little or no loss due to damage in transit. Supermarkets love the force-ripened tomatoes because they are virtually indestructible. They require no extra help or care. Even if they are handled like coal by careless employees or overzealous self-service shoppers, the supermarket tomatoes endure. Similar treatment to the vine-ripened kind would result in an almost immediate transformation to ketchup or tomato juice.

NUTRITIONAL DATA

One cup of tomato juice yields the following important nutrients: 8 mg. calcium, 29 mg. phosphorus, 0.59 mg. iron, 10 mg. sodium, 254 mg. potassium, 1,394 I.U. vitamin A, 2 mcg biotin, 11.5 mcg folic acid, 21.6 mg. vitamin C, and 14 mg. magnesium.

THERAPEUTIC BENEFITS

The introduction of the tomato into the early American diet as a useful food and helpful medicine was largely due to the efforts of a 19th-century "yankee huckster of the first class" as the great American historian Hubert Howe Bancroft described him in his book, *History of Utah* (San Francisco: The History Co., 1889; pp. 149–50). His name was Dr. John Cook Bennett.

He was appointed President of the medical department of Willoughby University at Lake Erie in Chagrin, Ohio. In his opening lecture in November 1834, Bennett was one of the first individuals to report that tomatoes successfully treated diarrhea, violent bilious attacks, dyspepsia (indigestion), prevented cholera, and restored the integrity of the liver to its original state of health. He resigned his position in March 1835 and commenced an active campaign all through the Western Reserve in behalf of the wonderful "magical tomato." Bennett's views were reprinted for decades in medical journals, newspapers, and gardening and agricultural periodicals, not only in the U.S., but also in Australia, the United Kingdom, and France.

Historian Bancroft aptly characterized Bennett this way: "He has ability, he has brains and fingers; but he has *no soul!*" However, the man without a soul knew enough about tomatoes, at a time when most Americans still regarded them as poisonous fruit, to know that they were excellent nourishment for weak livers.

About 120 years later a Japanese scientist working out of Tohoku University in Sendai, Japan published an important paper corroborating just about everything that Bennett had claimed. In *The Tohoku Journal of Experimental Medicine* (57:343–48, 1953) Dr. Yumi Tohuoka reported that "fresh tomato juice . . . was very effective in accelerating the glycogen [sugar] formation" in the livers of normal rabbits. Also, when the normal function of the liver was temporarily disturbed by different chemical agents, tomato juice caused the liver to immediately rebound from such a relapse. His conclusion was "that tomato is effective clinically in improving liver disturbance."

Based on Bennett's early claims, Dr. Tohuoka's investigations, and my own personal observations over two decades with hundreds of liver cases that I've consulted, *nothing* works better for improving the health and state of the liver *promptly* than does ordinary tomato juice! It is, quite literally, a bugle call to awaken the liver from any lethargy it might be in. For any energy-draining diseases such as hypoglycemia, chronic fatigue syndrome, yeast infection, and mononucleosis, tomato or low-sodium V-8® juice is where it's at for feeling great in a matter of minutes!

Tomato juice is terrific for any health problems that may drain body energy levels. However, for about 20 percent of rheumatoid arthritis victims it may prove to be aggravating and actually increase their pain and swelling further; so they would be better off leaving it alone.

Chronic Fatigue Syndrome, Fatigue, Hypoglycemia, Yeast Infection. All of these health problems have one thing in common— they drain the body's energy reserves and leave it mostly in a weakened state. Tomato juice with a pinch of cayenne pepper and dash of hot sauce added, well stirred, and completely drunk will revitalize the liver and adrenal glands within half-an-hour and prove a feeling of vitality which should last for several hours.

Appetite (Poor). An organically grown, vine-ripened tomato always has an alkaline smell and taste to it. This is because the fruit is very rich in mineral salts, which create an appetite soon after being consumed. These minerals also stimulate the flow of saliva, which adds to the feeling of hunger and enables food to be digested better. Juice made from such properly raised tomatoes and taken internally will help to get rid of eating disorders such as anorexia.

METHOD OF PREPARATION

Tomatoes are easy to juice. Wash them off, cut them into quarter sections, and juice. If using supermarket tomatoes in a Vita-Mix, I'd add a cup of water to make extra juice. Canned or bottled tomato juice or low-sodium V-8® juice work just as well. Season with a pinch of cayenne pepper and a drizzle of lime or lemon juice for added flavor.

WATERCRESS-TURNIP JUICES

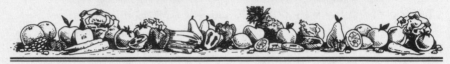

"Dynamic Drink for Fighting Infections"

DESCRIPTION

Watercress (*Nasturtium officinale*) carries its small, round, pungent leaves on long petioles from a much-branched stem that sprawls over the bottom of clear, shallow streams or in wet, shady places. It is a perennial of northern climates, and can live as long as the water doesn't freeze solid. It is quite similar to the mustard leaf in pungency, and sweeter than highland cress, which makes it very much in demand as a salad plant. The tender stems as well as the leaves are used.

In Great Britain it has been extremely popular for many decades with afternoon tea. The sharp, peppery flavor of the watercress sandwiches complements the delicate nip of the hot English tea. Watercress is very perishable. Only that which looks very green and fresh should be purchased, put into a plastic bag and sealed, and then put into your refrigerator and used within a few days.

The turnip (*Brassica rapa*) is a native of northeastern Europe. Turnips and rutabagas are closely related. When planted in the garden in the spring, it is an annual that sends up a tall, much-branched flowering stalk with pale-lavender flowers and long, slender, cylindrical pointed pods. When the seed is planted late in the season, it is a winter annual, as it doesn't send up the seedstalk until the following spring.

Turnips come in round, flat, or top shapes, and one variety is actually cylindrical in shape. Regardless of the variety, all turnips have the same flavor if grown under the same conditions. In the South turnips are widely grown for their delicious green tops; turnip greens is a mainstay for many a fine Southern meal. The root is as colorful as any fresh fruit. It is something like a beet, smooth-skinned, and pure white in color, with a royal purple crown. If they weren't so plentiful, turnips might pass for an exotic vegetable and command high market prices.

Choose only attractive-looking, colorful, firm, fresh white turnips that are heavy in relation to size. The smaller ones will have a much better flavor and texture than the larger ones. Avoid any that are misshapen, discolored, or soft. A sprouting at the crown end of the topless turnip is a sign of age or improper storage; such should be avoided as they don't taste good eaten raw and make lousy juice.

NUTRITIONAL DATA

One cup of fresh watercress yields the following nutrients: 53 mg. calcium, 19 mg. phosphorus, 0.6 mg. iron, 18 mg. sodium, 99 mg. potassium, 1,720 I.U. vitamin A, 28 mg. vitamin C, and 6.5 mg. magnesium. One-third of watercress is pure sulphur!

One cup of diced turnips contains: 51 mg. calcium, 39 mg. phosphorus, 0.7 mg. iron, 64 mg. sodium, 348 mg. potassium, trace of vitamin A, 47 mg. vitamin C, and 25 mg. magnesium.

THERAPEUTIC BENEFITS

Jan van der Hooven is a Dutch molecular biologist and immunologist residing in the city of Bergen op Zoom in the Netherlands. In the middle of October, 1993 we corresponded together on separate research that each of us has been doing in regard to sulphur fruits and vegetable. Dr. van der Hooven shared with me an item of his own recent discovery: sulphur- and potassium-rich vegetables exhibit positive influences in the bodies of those individuals afflicted with various sexually transmissible diseases and tuberculosis.

Grateful for the information, I decided to put it to the test the first opportunity I got. I didn't have to wait very long. Vincent Grolier of Chevy Chase, Maryland wrote to ask what he could do for a promiscuous friend of his who had contracted chlamydia, an infectious sexually transmissible disease. His friend experienced frequent pain and discomfort in the urinary and genital tracts and painful urination.

I advised him to have his friend drink a combination of watercress-turnip juice twice a day. The high sulphur content in watercress would help to kill the viruses causing his friend's chlamydia, and the turnip juice would make the other more palatable to drink. In just seven weeks, he reported back that "my friend is 'cured' thanks to your recommendation."

The second instance to put Dr. van der Hooven's discovery to the test came right here in my own back yard. A young local doctor with an open mind and good attitude was treating a Vietnam War vet suffering from tuberculosis at the Salt Lake City Veteran's Administration Hospital. Nothing in his regular arsenal of drugs seemed to be helping much. He happened to tune in late one morning to the Bob Lee Show on KSL Radio, and heard me discussing the usual foods and herbs for this-and-that diseases which people called in with seeking answers for.

Because the lines were jammed, he couldn't get through any of the studio phones, but left his number for me to call him after the show was over. We had an amiable chat and he said how much he enjoyed the show. He then told me about this particular case for which nothing pharmaceutical seemed to be working. I recommended the watercress-turnip juice combination again. He asked if he could get them in powdered forms to give his patient, thinking that would be a lot easier. I told him "good luck" if he could find such, because then he'd know something that I didn't know. I suggested that he invest in a good juicer, told him how to prepare the mixture, and to give his patient two small glasses of this every day with meals. He said he would have to make the juice at home and then bring it to the hospital and give it to the man without any of his colleagues seeing it.

Sometime later, I got a call in my other office in South Salt Lake at the monthly seniors newspaper I've been editor of now for a couple of years. It was my friend from the VA Hospital. He congratulated me on "something that worked, even to my own astonishment." He said the addition of the liquid Kyolic garlic to the juice mix, undoubtedly was of "great benefit" for this patient, too. (I had neglected to mention this earlier.) He wondered what it was, though, in these three items that had made such remarkable improvement in a very stubborn case of drug-resistant TB. I told him, quite plainly, it was the sulphur compounds in the watercress and Kyolic garlic that did the trick.

Asthma, Bronchitis, Emphysema, Pneumonia, Whooping Cough. The following popular European remedy has been used for a number of respiratory disorders in England, France, and Germany. Take equal parts (2 tablespoons) of watercress and turnip juices, goat milk, and dark honey. Mix together in a tin cup, briefly heat over a flame until warm, and then take internally by spoon. Repeat every several hours as needed.

Abscesses, Boils, Cankers, Carbuncles, Whitlows. Sterilize a sewing needle over a flame and then lance the skin eruption. Take a 4 inch square piece of layered cheesecloth and soak it in some watercress juice. Wring out excess liquid. Place into the center of it a small half spoonful of turnip pulp and spread out evenly. Apply directly to the skin, cover with another layered cheesecloth of the same dimensions and hold in place with your hand or some tape. Repeat with another dressing 30 minutes later. Do this three times daily for several days until all of the purulent matter has been drawn out.

METHOD OF PREPARATION

Separate a small bunch of watercress and wash it under running water in a metal or plastic colander that you might use for draining cooked spaghetti noodles in. Add a cup of water to your Vita-Mix and juice the watercress. Then wash and cube a medium-sized turnip and juice it as well *with* the watercress juice still in the container. Divide into two equal portions and drink eight hours apart with meals.

WATERMELON JUICE

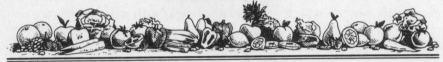

"Native American Recovery Program for Illness"

DESCRIPTION

It is believed by some ethnologists (scientists who study different cultures) that the watermelon (*Citrullus vulgaris*) was first introduced among the Hopi by the arrival of the Spanish friars to the American Southwest sometime in the mid-1600s. Since the Hopis didn't have horses at that time, but the Spaniards did, this tribe gave the nickname of "horse pumpkins" to this new vegetable-fruit. The early Hopi claimed that a fresh watermelon smelled like one of the sweating horses that their foreign visitors rode, according to Alfred Whiting in his book, *Ethnobotany of the Hopi* (Flagstaff: Northland Press, 1966; p. 93). Hence, the odd nickname for one of the principal food staples of several Southwestern Native American tribes.

It wasn't too long before watermelons were being planted everywhere in this region of country. The Jesuit priest Father Kino wrote in October 1700 that the Yumans he had visited had watermelons, and the Anza expeditions in the fall of 1775 recorded that the Yumans offered them an estimated three thousand watermelons, some being as big in size as a normal five-year-old child! (Edward

Castetter and Willis H. Bell. *Yuman Indian Agriculture* (Albuquerque: University of New Mexico Press, 1951; p. 129.)

All of the Southwest Indian tribes seemed to grow at least two different types of watermelons—one with pink seeds and yellow flesh and one with black seeds and yellow flesh. The normal watermelon is a trailing vine with deeply lobed, medium-sized leaves and yellow flowers which are borne in the axils of the leaves. The fruit ranges in size from a large grapefruit to a large field pumpkin *or bigger* sometimes, while the shape is anything from oval to cylindrical. The color is light or dark green, with gray-green stripes running lengthwise in some varieties.

Stone mountain is the watermelon most of us are well acquainted with. It is a large, oval, grayish-green melon with deep-crimson flesh and white seeds and matures in 88 days. The luscious golden sweet and a closely related type are what the Southwest tribes prefer. Both varieties are medium-large, longer than broad, with a golden-yellow flesh and dark-green rind. They require 83 days to mature.

The Southwest tribes have always highly valued their watermelons. The early varieties had very good storage qualities and could be packed in weeds and sand or hung in yucca fiber slings for storage until as late as February of the following year after being harvested in August. This was an important source of fresh food during the long, cold winter months. Among the Pueblo groups, watermelons were often given as gifts on ceremonial occasions.

Prior to cutting open a watermelon, it is next to impossible to judge its stage of maturity. Professional produce buyers will never buy a load of watermelon without cutting several random samples. These melons do ripen after being severed from the vine. The length of time that has elapsed since harvesting can be determined by the condition of the pigtail stem. When you purchase a watermelon, if the stem is fresh and green, the melon is probably too immature to cut and needs a few more days of ripening. After a few days the stem will shrink and discolor but will still be attached to the watermelon. This is a sign that the watermelon has reached the desired maturity. After another few days, the pigtail stem will part from the watermelon. A tailless watermelon may be overripe.

Forget about thumping a watermelon as evidence of its ripeness; this is only an exercise in futility. The only foolproof way to

judge the ripeness and the texture of a watermelon is to cut it open.
Retail markets sell cut watermelons by quarters and halves. Purchasing a whole uncut watermelon is sort of like buying the proverbial
"pig in a poke." Buying a quarter or a half is better for checking out
the color and flavor.

The perfect watermelon will have a firm, dark red flesh. If the
flesh is pale and pink, it isn't quite ripe and will lack sweetness. If
the flesh is soft or shattered, the melon is overripe and will have a
lousy taste and texture. Even in a perfect watermelon, the blossom-
end half is always slightly riper and sweeter than the stem-end half.

NUTRITIONAL DATA

One cup of diced watermelon pieces contains: 11 mg. calcium, 16
mg. phosphorus, 0.8 mg. iron, 2 mg. sodium, 160 mg. potassium, 940
I.U. vitamin A, 11 mg. vitamin C, 3.4 mcg folic acid, 17 mg.
magnesium, and 0.11 mg. zinc.

THERAPEUTIC BENEFITS

Ethnologist Leslie Spier, in his book, *Yuman Tribes of the Gila River*
(Chicago: University of Chicago Press, 1933; p. 65), made reference
to the use of watermelon juice by some Southwest Indian groups.
Tribal women, he reported, would squeeze the fresh watermelon
pulp between their hands to get all of the juice out, after which the
juice was strained through muslin cloth into another pan and then
boiled into a syrup.

Anthropologist Daryll C. Ford reported in 1931 that while
watermelon were planted and cultivated by the men of different
households, it was their women who owned the fields in which they
were grown. He related how the women from Shongopavi, one of
several Hopi villages, employed this watermelon juice syrup for a
variety of pulmonary disorders, gastrointestinal complaints, skin
problems, and major organ dysfunctions. (Daryll C. Forde, "Hopi
Agriculture and Land Ownership." *Journal of the Royal Anthropological Institute of Great Britain and Ireland* 61:357–405, 1931.)

My own research conducted at Old Oraibi well over a decade
ago confirms the value of watermelon juice in helping a weak and

enfeebled system fully recuperate from recent illness or surgery. The village of Old Oraibi is situated on the edge of a lonely mesa north of Winslow, Arizona. It is the oldest continuously inhabited townsite in North America, being built in 1150 A.D. and, still as of the end of 1993, containing a few remaining occupants. My Hopi informant then, an old, wrinkled, toothless woman of the Patki clan told how she had used fresh squeezed melon juice in times past for curing fevers, stopping the colic in young babies, getting rid of sour stomachs from "eating too much of the white man's food," relieving headaches, and giving energy and strength where needed in the some of the elderly folks. She maintained that she still was able to get around pretty well, thanks in part to watermelons!

Arthritis, Gout, Uremic Poisoning. This trio of afflictions share one thing in common—an excess accumulation of uric acid. Glasses of fresh watermelon juice (minus the seeds) morning and evening will help to flush such poison out of the body.

Skin Problems. Eruptions on the surface of the skin usually indicate an acidic condition in the blood. This comes from eating too much meat, fried food, sweets, and white flour products, as well as drinking a lot of coffee, colas, and soft drinks. Watermelon juice flushes a lot of this acid from the system and renews the blood. When this happens the skin starts looking and feeling better.

METHOD OF PREPARATION

Cut the ripe flesh from the watermelons and juice in your juicing machine. No water needs to be added as it will make plenty of its own juice. Then pour through a wire strainer to remove the seeds and drink one small glass twice daily as needed for rejuvenating the system.

The Mojaves, Yumas, Cocopas, and Maricopas have all consumed watermelon seeds whole after they've been parched. They would eat them like pinenuts. Sometimes the oily meal was mixed with mesquite flour. The seeds were also boiled sometimes and the tea drunk for uro-genital complaints. (Castetter and Bell, *op. cit.*)

WHEAT GRASS–BARLEY GRASS JUICES

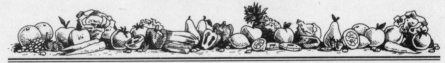

"A Renewal of Life in Every Glass"

DESCRIPTION

There are two types of wheat grass. The first is the cereal plant of the genus *Triticum* of the grass family, and believed to have evolved from an ancient form of the seldom cultivated einkorn species. It is a major food and an important commodity on the world grain market. Modern wheat varieties are usually classified as winter wheats (fall-planted and unusually winter hardy for grain crops) and spring wheats. Roughly three-quarters of the wheat grown in the U.S. today is winter wheat (*Triticum aestivum*). When in its young grass stage, the wheat plant is harvested and this wheat grass is used for eating and juicing purposes.

The second type of wheat grass is any plant of the *Agropyron* genus. These cool-season perennials belonging to the same grass family are important range forage in the prairie states. They are also valuable for revegetation because of their drought reistance and winter hardiness. Quack grass belongs to this group. While good for hungry cattle, they make lousy juice and can actually aggravate existing allergies.

Barley (*Hordeum vulgare*) is also an annual cereal grass of the same family as wheat. It was known to the ancient Greeks, Romans, Chinese, and Egyptians and was the chief bread material in Europe as late as the 16th century. It has a wide range of cultivation and matures even at high altitudes, since its growing season is so short; but, it can't withstand hot and humid climates. The ancients made some great brews from their barley harvests, and a few of those fantastic recipes have managed to survive for several thousand years. I've tasted Sumerian beer brewed from barley exactly as it was back in 2550 B.C. It reminded me of an English mead or ale, only more flavorful and with full-body to it. Compared to this elegant brew, most American beers taste like dishwater!!

Today barley is typically a special-purpose grain with many different varieties rather than just a general market crop like wheat. It is a valuable stock feed (often used as a corn substitute) and is used for malting when the grain is of high quality. It is a minor source of flour and breakfast foods. Pearl barley is often used in soups. In the Middle East, a limited amount of barley is eaten like rice. In the U.S. most spring barley comes from the western states and most winter barley is grown in the southeastern states for fall and spring pasture and as a cover crop.

Like winter wheat, barley is also planted in the fall and is grown for approximately 200 days through the winter in the Great Plains of the United States and the prairie provinces of Canada. It is harvested in the spring just prior to "jointing." The jointing stage is that point at which the internodal tissue in wheat or barley leaves begin to elongate, forming stems. This stage represents the peak of their vegetative development. This is when they should be mechanically cut and juiced.

NUTRITIONAL DATA

I am indebted to my friend Ronald L. Seibold of Pines International, an American-owned and operated cereal grass juice manufacturer in Lawrence, Kansas for the following data. It comes from an excellent book he edited and helped fund, entitled *Cereal Grass: What's In It For You!* (Lawrence, KS: Wilderness Community Education Foundation, 1990).

The following nutritional analysis is typical of dehydrated cereal grass. The nutrients represent 3.5 grams of substance, which is the equivalent of seven 500 mg. tablets or one teaspoonful of powdered cereal grass. They are as follows: 1,750 I.U. vitamin A, 280 mcg vitamin K, 11 mg. vitamin C, 1.1 mcg vitamin E, 10 mcg thiamin, 1 mg. choline, 71 mcg riboflavin, 45 mcg pyridoxine, 1 mcg vitamin B-12, 263 mcg niacin, 84 mcg pantothenic acid, 4 mcg biotin, 38 mcg folic acid, 18 mg. calcium and phosphorus, 112 mg. potassium, 3.6 mg. magnesium, 2 mg. iron, 0.35 mg. manganese, 3.5 mcg selenium, 1 mg. sodium, 17.5 mcg zinc, 7 mcg iodine, 0.02 mg. copper, and 1.75 mcg cobalt. Total protein is 800 mg, crude fiber 600 mg., calories 10, chlorophyll 19 mg. and carbohydrates 1.3 grams. Cereal grass powder has 20 essential and non-essential amino acids. Five grams (0.175 oz) of dehydrated cereal grass yields more grams of fiber per serving than does equivalent amounts of oat bran and cooked whole wheat cereal. It is nearly equal to equivalent amounts of wheat bran and prunes in total dietary fiber. (This data was taken from tables on pages 51 and 53 of the aforementioned book. Copies of this excellent study are available at $13.95 (postage included) from Pines Int'l. See Appendix Three for details.)

THERAPEUTIC BENEFITS

In the mid-to-late 1930s, dairy scientists at the University of Wisconsin noticed that the nutritional value of summer milk was much higher than that of cow's milk produced at other seasons of the year. When fed on summer milk, experimental lab animals thrived, but when it was replaced with winter milk they eventually became sick and died. Scientists accounted for the nutritional difference in each seasonal milk to the enriching meadow and cereal grasses the cows had free access to during the summer months. Thus began intensive research into what later became known as the "grass juice factor."

During the social upheavals and environmental turbulence of the 1960s and 70s, Ann Wigmore began her own research on cereal grasses and cereal grass juices. She had witnessed first-hand her own grandmother curing injured soldiers during World War I with wheat and barley grass and believed there was, indeed, some healing value to them.

Ann started chewing young blades of wheat grass which grew near her house. Soon she found it much easier to drink the juice instead. It wasn't too long before she got over her colitis. She then began giving some juice to her dogs and cats, with amazing results. Like her, they became more active and peppy, and showed unbounded energy.

Word of these small health miracles soon spread to some of her surrounding sick friends and neighbors. They began to ask her for some of this "magical potion or elixir." Upon receiving and drinking the same in copious amounts, many of them, she relates, "got right up out of their sick beds, much to the amazement of relatives and doctors, and went on about their business as if nothing had ever happened to them!"

In 1968 Ann founded the Hippocrates Health Institute in Boston, Massachusetts. It soon became the country's leading health treatment and education center. Her mainstays for treating many chronic degenerative diseases were wheat grass and barley grass juices, along with a raw foods diet. Because she wasn't a doctor, nor had a medical license to practice, the thousands who visited her over the next few decades, came as her specially invited "guests" and basically stayed for free. Private donations were given "under the counter, around the corner, and sometimes over the roof," Ann is fond of recalling with a mischievous twinkle in her clear eyes.

"I even cured the so-called 'incurables,'" she boasts. The doctors would send me their near-dead or dying cancer patients, telling them in advance, 'We've done everything medically possible for you in the way of surgery, radiation, and chemotherapy. Now we're going to turn you over to this woman, so that if you die, you'll at least die of quackery and not by our hands or methods.' The people who crawled, barely walked, or had to be carried in, somehow seemed to survive even by the slimmest of margins. They got well and lived to tell or write about it!" Such as Eydie Maie Hunsberger, who wrote *How I Conquered Cancer Naturally!*

Ann believes that wheat and barley grass juice are good for any number of ailments, which are mentioned in the final section of this particular entry. Others have done similar work with juices, such as Viktoras Kulvinskas and the Japanese research pharmacist Yoshihide Hagiwara. No one has done what Ann has done, in pioneering the use of both cereal grass juices for so many different diseases.

There are others like Charlotte Gerson, who has carried on the work of her father, Max Gerson, M.D. at the Centro Hospitalario International del Pacifico (CHIPSA) in Tijuana, Mexico but despite all of the wonderful things which she and her staff have been able to achieve with their own numerous sick patients over the years, neither cereal grass has figured into her particular regimen.

I had an opportunity to interview both Ann Wigmore and her recovered cancer patient Eydie Mae Hunsberger at the Health & Fitness Expo held in the Syria Mosque on Fifth & Bigelow in Pittsburgh Saturday and Sunday, April 16–17, 1983. To this date I can still see the ruddy-cheeked octogenarian hurrying around her crowded hotel room to find her various wheat and barley grass trays which she had packed with her. I watched as she placed her worn out juicer on top of the bathroom counter and plugged it into the wall outlet intended mainly for electric razors. As she clipped her five-day cereal grass sprouts and tossed handfuls into the container, I casually remarked, "You do go to *a lot* of trouble to juice them, don't you?"

Without ever taking her eyes off of what she was doing, she responded, "Yes, but just look at how much the trouble has been worth — an 80-year-old granny in the body of a 35-year-old woman!" Even by my own picky standards of feminine beauty, she wasn't all that bad-looking, considering the incredible expanses of age involved.

Eydie was more to the point, when I spoke with her next. "The doctors offered me no life, no hope, nothing to live for. Only death, death, death! I thought, what do I have to lose by going to this woman whom the medics labelled as 'an old crazy quack.' At least I'll be dying with some dignity to me. But Ann's juice therapy offered me more than hope or empty dreams. It *gave me* MY LIFE back again! A new lease on life! Or better still…*A RENEWAL OF LIFE* I never imagined possible, considering the horrible state of health I was in at the time."

Alcoholism.   Alcohol wrecks the liver. Cereal grasses are rich in mineral salts and dark chlorophyll, which help to rejuvenate the liver by repairing some of the damage done.

Drug Addiction.   The high calcium, magnesium, phosphorus, and potassium salts in cereal grasses flush out drug residues from organs and muscle tissue.

Fatigue. The solution to a lack of energy doesn't lay in sweet things, but rather in chlorophyll-rich foods. Cereal grass juices are high in vitamins, minerals, and enzymes, which have a dynamic effect upon the liver. When this happens it creates more energy within the body.

Infections. Chlorophyll has a powerful effect on infectious diseases. The abundant vitamin A and C contents of cereal grasses enhance the performance of the immune system dramatically. When this takes place, problems ranging from cancers to colds begin to go into remission.

Malnutrition. Those suffering from extreme hunger for sustained periods of time will benefit immensely from cereal grass juices. However, care needs to be taken when they are being given this. Wheat grass and barley grass juices should always be mixed with some other type of juice, so as to reduce flatulence. These juices need to be given in small, measured doses so as not to overwhelm an extremely weakened system.

METHOD OF PREPARATION

Indoor, tray-grown wheat or barley grasses that send up shoots in a week or less, are still quite popular among sprouting enthusiasts. As Ron Seibold once explained to me (and amply does so in his book, too), such will never reach the important jointing stage where their simple sugars can be converted to the complex nutrients that field-grown wheat or barley grasses contain. That's why tray-grown cereal grasses have such a strong sweet taste and in large amounts can make a person feel nauseous and sick. It takes prairie soil, cold weather, fall planting, *slow* winter growth, and early spring harvest to make the ideal cereal grasses.

These are available in concentrated juice powders, which saves time, effort, and money to make. Besides those which Ron's company sells, there is also an outstanding product made by Wakunaga of America. It is called Kyo-Green and is available in health food stores nationwide (see Appendix Three for details). Of all the cereal grass juices on the market, it is, by far, the most complete I believe. It consists of the concentrated juices from young wheat and barley grasses, an algae called chlorella, the seaweed kelp, and brown rice.

The ULTIMATE health juice cocktail I routinely prescribe for others and take plenty of myself is made from the following ingredients: one level tablespoonful Kyo-Green; one teaspoonful liquid Kyolic aged garlic extract; one level teaspoonful Pines' organic beet juice powder; and 10 fluid ounces of pure spring water. Blend it quickly for 15 seconds in your Vita-Mix and drink straight. It gives the body life and vitality for the rest of the day!

ZUCCHINI SQUASH JUICE

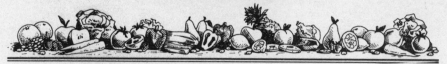

"Incredible Energy for Chronic Fatigue Syndrome"

DESCRIPTION

Zucchini squash, it will be observed, has the same Latin binomial (*Cucurbita pepo*) as does pumpkin, showing that it is really a bush pumpkin instead of a squash. The green zucchini fruits are usually three times as long as broad, cylindrical in shape, and have a light gray mottled effect.

At one time the green-skinned zucchini was a rarity in produce markets and could only be found in retail stores in large Italian neighborhoods. It slowly gained in popularity, until today it is the biggest seller of the bush pumpkin group. As an example, consider the summer squash sales at New York's Point Market place: 95% of what is sold each year is zucchini.

Zucchini is of definite Italian origin as the name implies. In French restaurants and British cookbooks it's referred to as *courgette*, while in other places it is simply called green squash.

The unopened flower buds of zucchini are a gourmet item. When they are sauteed they are a great flavor treat. These buds are very expensive when bought in fancy produce shops, but are free for the taking if you grow your own zucchini.

smaller the seed, the better the flavor and the smoother the texture. The smaller the squash, the smaller the seeds. Therefore, the smaller zucchini (about seven inches in length) and the firmer, the better it is.

Zucchini

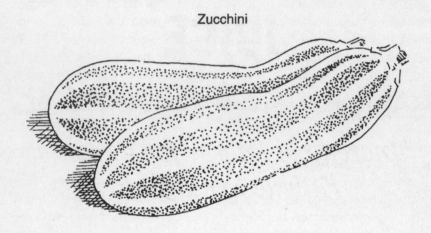

NUTRITIONAL DATA

One cup of raw, sliced zucchini squash yields the following important nutrients: 36 mg. calcium, 38 mg. phosphorus, 0.5 mg. iron, 11 mg. sodium, 263 mg. potassium, 530 I.U. vitamin A, 1.3 mg. niacin, 29 mg. vitamin C, and 21 mg. magnesium.

The late physician to some of the old Hollywood movie stars, Henry G. Bieler, M.D., declared in his national bestseller *Food Is Your Best Medicine* (New York: Random House, 1966; p. 204) "that the zucchini is an especially sodium-rich vegetable." Organic sodium, he insisted, "is the most ideal source of refurbishing a sodium-exhausted liver."

THERAPEUTIC BENEFITS

Some of Hollywood's great and not-so-great talents were treated at various times in their lives by Dr. Bieler. Said the late and mysterious

Greta Garbo: "I had known Dr. Bieler for a great many years. He helped me through a crisis by prescribing the right types of food." Hedda Hopper, the film gossip columnist, once wrote: "I've known this man for 25 years and if I'd always taken his advice like I should have, I'd never have had a sick day during all that time."

It was the late screen actress Gloria Swanson, who offered personal testimony concerning Dr. Bieler's food therapy prescriptions. I met this aging film star some years ago at a large holistic health conference in Los Angeles, where she had a small speaking part in one of the sessions. We were introduced to each other via a mutual friend.

After an exchange of the usual politesse and some general small talk, the conversation became more meaningful when she related something from her past that she said I could use, but only after agreeing to do so when she passed on.

She began to feel very weak for no apparent reason. This physical weakness came on quite suddenly. It worried her quite a bit. But what concerned her the most was even why it should have happened, since she was known to follow a natural foods diet pretty closely anyway.

She made an appointment to see Dr. Bieler. He gave her a thorough physical checkup and ran some blood and urine tests for a sugar count. He informed Ms. Swanson that her blood sugar was extremely low. This baffled her and she explained to him that she consumed a wide variety of fresh fruits.

Much to her surprise, he told her that this was the cause of her problem; and told her to lay off the fruits and fruit juices for a while. He recommended that she eat cooked zucchini squash instead, and also drink the raw zucchini juice every day, one cup with a meal.

Ms. Swanson followed his advice, admitting to me, however, that "it was the hardest thing that I have ever done in my life. The craving for fruits simply would not go away. I found the urge to sneak some grapes or eat an orange, was almost irresistible." After being on the good doctor's peculiar diet for several weeks, "suddenly my fatigue disappeared one morning, and I awoke with the energy I used to have. I was so happy I could have kissed the man (meaning Dr. Bieler)." This is an incredible true testimony of the wonderful effects which zucchini juice can have on a weak liver!

Calcium Malabsorption, Osteoporosis.   Zucchini juice contains enough chelated calcium to be retained in the body longer than dairy or food supplement calcium. This tends to strengthen weak bones and prevents them from becoming brittle.

Fractures, Bone Breaks.   Zuchinni juice is remarkable for the way it can help to knit bones together in a shorter period of time. The calcium, phosphorus, magnesium, and sodium are all about equally balanced in content amounts. With the strong presence of potassium, they are able to do such mending incredibly sooner than it would take with individual food supplements of each of these minerals.

METHOD OF PREPARATION

You won't find zucchini juice covered in any juicing books that I know of. I've checked ten of them out so far, and unless I've missed something, they just don't make mention of this vegetable at all. Based on the miraculous experiences of some of the former patients of the late Dr. Bieler, I started recommending this juice myself to others who suffer from chronic fatigue syndrome.

I instruct them to wash a zucchini under running water, but *never* to peel it. I advise cutting it lengthwise several times, and then crosswise into little pieces, which juice easier in a Vita-Mix. One-half to a whole cup of water may need to be added to liquefy things more. One-half cup should then be drunk with every meal, or else mixed in with an equal amount of tomato or carrot juice to improve the flavor.

APPENDIX ONE

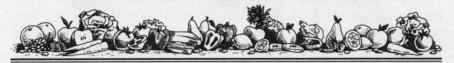

Setting Up Your Own Home Juice Bar

PICKING THE RIGHT JUICER

There are basically three different ways to obtain juice from fruits and vegetables. The first is as old a method as humanity itself. This is the manual operation of squeezing something by one or both hands in order to get out every drop of juice possible. For some items such as berries or citrus fruits, this is a fairly easy task. For other things like melons or cucumbers, it is going to be more difficult but not impossible. However, unless you possess the strength of Superman you'll not get very far squeezing a carrot, radish, potato, or celery stalk by hand. The only aggravations you'll reap are a sore hand and wrist, a dislocated thumb, or carpel tunnel syndrome.

The second method is to invest in some kind of juicing machine. There are two basic types: centrifugal and masticating. In a centrifugal juicer, fruits and vegetables are finely chopped up in a plastic or stainless steel basket, before being spun at a terrific rate of speed to separate the juice from the pulp. The juice pours out of a spigot and the pulp stays in the machine. Another version of this type of juicer includes a pulp ejector, which throws out the pulp after the juice has come through first. The masticating juicer grinds whatever produce is inserted into a mealy paste before spinning it very rapidly to squeeze the juice through a screen set into the machine bottom.

There are several nutritional drawbacks to this method of juicing. The most obvious is that the pulp is entirely discarded. Numerous medical studies have shown that fiber is an essential part of human health; and without adequate fiber in the diet, a person can become susceptible to a whole host of degenerative diseases. The second, less obvious, problem is with the blood sugar imbalances that are created by drinking straight juice *without* the fiber. With some juices this isn't that critical, but with others high in natural sugar contents, this can be very troublesome, especially if a person is already afflicted with diabetes or hypoglycemia, the two most common blood sugar disorders around.

Drinking *pure* apple, carrot, grape, or orange juices minus their fiber, wreaks havoc with the body's own blood sugar levels. It is tantamount to driving a car without adequate brakes. In order for such a vehicle to be safely operational, it must have a good braking system. The pulp of naturally sweet fruits and vegetables is the very mechanism by which their sugar contents are more *slowly* assimilated into the body rather than rapidly so. When using any kind of juicer that discards the pulp, you are essentially doing away with the built-in safety mechanism that would prevent a sudden "sugar overload" from occurring in your body. Furthermore, without the accompanying fiber, the sweet fruit or vegetable juices you might be drinking will have quite a "yo-yo effect" on your system.

To prevent havoc being played with your blood sugar levels, therefore, you need to consider the third and most reasonable option in juicing. That is what I call the "puree juicing" method. For this you need a unique piece of equipment I like to designate as "a blender juicer." Unlike true juicers such as the centrifugal or masticating kinds which separate the pulp from the produce, a "blender juicer" purees everything—pulp, skin, and seeds. Another way of looking at it is to say that a "blender juicer" keeps the brakes on the car in order to prevent a blood sugar accident from occurring down the road.

Prevention Health Magazine's Food Center and Test Kitchen decided to conduct an informal demonstration and taste test using three of the top juicers on the market representing the three different methods of juicing. For centrifugal, they chose an Omega, for mastication, a Champion juicer, and for what I've termed "puree juicing," they picked a Vita-Mix Total Nutrition Center unit. Each juicer was individually tested, following manufacturers' specific directions, three different times. Every time, the testers processed foods of distinctly different densities: carrots, pineapples, and tomatoes. They also noted each juicer's ease of assembly, operation, and cleanup. Their final results were published in the January, 1993 issue of *Prevention* magazine (pp. 61–64) under the rather auspicious heading "A Consumer's Guide to Juice—and Juicers."

Here is a brief run-down on the conclusions they drew regarding each juicer.

The Omega grated the food, then extracted the juice by means of centrifugal force. Produce was pressed against a rotating wheel of fine blades at the base of a sievelike basket. The grated material was then flung against the sieve, with the juice filtering through afterwards. Taste-testers gave high ratings for the carrot and pineapple juices it produced, but were very disappointed with the "thick and frothy" tomato juice. Cleanup was, indeed, a chore. They had to unscrew the clutch nut that held the blade and dismantled the pulp-catching cylindrical strainer from the bowl. The pulp had to be scraped out by hand. The bowl, basket and blade parts were then rinsed with cool water only—never with hot water and never in a dishwasher! For those who like screwing and unscrewing things, and cleaning a lot with their hands, they may contact: Omega Products, 6291 Lyters Lane, POB 4523, Harrisburg, PA 17111.

The Champion finely chewed the produce put into it before extruding the juice from the pulp via hydraulic pressure. Because there are 4 to 5 individual pieces that need assembling and disassembling every time you juice, it can become rather burdensome and time-consuming. Also you need to get your own bowls to collect the juice and pulp in or else face a big mess on your kitchen counter top and floor. The items juiced ranked from pretty high for taste, except the pineapple, which turned out quite soupy and resembled canned pineapple juice. Cleanup was anything but a breeze. It took patience and time to take everything apart, scrub it by hand in cold, soapy water, and then rinse before drying. No parts of this juicer are dishwasher-safe at all. For those into frequent assembling/disassembling of major components and who don't mind getting rough, dishwasher hands, they can write to: Plastaket Manufacturing Co., Inc., 6220 East Highway 12 (Victor Rd.), Lodi, CA 95240.

Of the three juice machines tested, the *Prevention* magazine testing team reserved their loudest compliments and applause for the

Vita-Mix. For juicing, they wrote, "one machine stands head and motor above the rest: Vita-Mix!" They marvelled at how "user friendly" it was—practically no assembly required. They were equally ecstatic over the nice "smooth drinks chock-full of the fruit's original goodness and fiber" that the Vita-Mix produced every single time. They described how this machine "rose to the challenge" when "puree juicing" carrots. They warmly praised it as being "the most versatile of the juicers we tested. . ." So far as cleaning went, it was almost as easy as snapping your fingers! They filled the blenderlike container with hot, soapy water one time and put it back on the base and turned it on. Another time, they simply rinsed out the container and dome-shaped lid and set them on a drain board. The third time they put both container and lid upside down in their kitchen dishwasher to clean.

Even more precise testing with five different juicers was conducted by Wolf Technical Services of Aurora, Ohio. I received a copy of their Project Report No. 921002 (dated November 19, 1992) from which the following information was obtained. Five juicing machines were used in their test operations:

1. The Juiceman, Automatic Juice Extractor, Type 42.1 , Fab. Nr. 10-90 (Made in Poland).

2. The Juiceman II, Automatic Juice Extractor, Model TR-50C, S/N 1-1108266 (Made in Korea).

3. Olympic, Fruit and Vegetable Juicer, Model 100, S/N 05415 (Made in Penn. and Calif.).

4. The Champion, World's Finest Juicer, S/N Y-65839; equipped with a G.E. Model No. G5-NG-8535 Motor (Made in Calif.).

5. Vita-Mix, Maxi-4000, Model 479044, Commercial/Household Type (Made in Ohio).

Eight Ohio residents were selected to produce about $\frac{1}{2}$ gallon quantity of juice consisting of apples, oranges, pineapples, and bananas. Everything was carefully tabulated and the final data recorded on Table I of the technical report. Besides the obvious fact that there was *no* pulp waste with the Vita-Mix (as there was with the other machines), there was also considerable savings of time in the actual juicing and final cleanup.

The accompanying table shows the average amount of time recorded for each machine. Notice how quickly the Vita-Mix juiced and cleaned up afterwards compared to the other four machines.

Juice Machine	Processing Minutes	Clean-Up Minutes
Juiceman	*10.402*	*5.300*
Juiceman II	*4.972*	*5.673*
Champion	*12.742*	*6.651*
Olympic	*15.081*	*7.538*
Vita-Mix	*2.642*	*1.044*

So if you want a complete juice that's totally nutritious, quick and easy to fix, and from a machine that will save you time, then contact these folks: Vita-Mix Corp., Dept. HEHJ, 8615 Usher Rd., Cleveland, OH 44138; or call them toll-free at 1-(800)-VITAMIX (800-848-2649).

TIPS FOR BLENDER JUICING SUCCESS

Always be sure to scrub thoroughly those fruits and vegetables you intend to juice. If they're the leafy type, such as spinach or Romaine lettuce, then rinse them several times under running tap water. Be sure to wash well whatever it is you're juicing!

Peeling and pitting may be necessary on some items. By removing bitter peelings and seeds when occasion requires doing so, it can definitely improve the flavor of your juices.

As I mentioned earlier in the text, avoid mixing fruit and vegetable juices together. I am aware that most other juice books advocate this. However, I don't, for the simple reason that most vegetables are alkaline and high in mineral salts, while most fruits are acidic and contain a lot of natural sugars. The body processes alkaline foods one way, and handles acid foods another way. Also, minerals undergo a special chelation process within the body so they can be properly stored where needed the most. On the other hand, carbohydrates are converted to fuel and "burned" within the system to produce energy and strength. When mineral-rich vegetable and sweet fruit juices are mixed together, they often produce intestinal discomfort and chemical disturbance within the body. Just remember to *keep them separate!*

If you've never owned a juicer, then it might be practical to follow the juice recipes in the beginning. But as you become more familiar with juicing in your blender, you can feel free to experiment and go for new juice blends that are exciting and dynamic in color and taste and feel in your mouth.

This is the *only* juice book which contains very detailed information on each fruit and vegetable presented. I've given readers specific information on what to look for in getting the best-tasting juices possible.

Don't forget seasonings either! Unlike fruits and vegetables, which shouldn't be mixed, spices are intriguing and adventuresome to use. Go ahead and throw some garlic powder in with your carrot-spinach-tomato cocktail. How about a pinch of cayenne pepper in your tomato-watercress-radish delight? A sprinkle of Mrs. Dash or granulated kelp, along with some liquid Kyolic aged garlic extract, can really enliven an otherwise boring wheat grass/barley grass juice combination. I still haven't gotten over the delicious flavor that pinches of ground cardamom or cinnamon can bring to peach, pear, or pineapple juices, or a mixture of all three. By adding some fresh grated ginger or nutmeg to a papaya-guava- mango mix or any of them separately, you'll discover for yourself just how exotic spices like these can make such tropical fruit juices taste.

Also keep in mind that a Vita-Mix engages in "puree juicing," which means that in many instances you will have to add a little extra water in order to dilute things so they're easier to drink. Additionally, you may want to still "count the calories" if you're worried about an expansion of waist girth. While juices contain virtually no fat, their calories can add up pretty fast, especially so with tropical fruits.

Remember that while you may be retaining the fiber along with natural sugars in sweet juices, there is still a chance of upsetting your body's blood sugar levels if you suffer from diabetes or hypoglycemia. It's a good idea in such cases to sip only a small amount of a particularly sweet juice at any given time. Then, after a while you'll be able to tell whether or not your body is reacting adversely to whatever you drank.

Finally, it's important to realize that fresh juice, made and consumed the *same* day, is by far better for you than juice that is refrigerated and kept for several days.

APPENDIX TWO

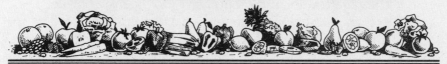

What To Do with the Leftover Pulp

When my esteemed colleague and long-time friend, retired pediatrician Lendon Smith, M.D. received a copy of the main text of this book and read it through to write the nice Foreword that appears in front, he didn't have the Appendices in hand at the time. When I spoke with him by phone towards the end of December, 1993 prior to receiving his Foreword, he had only legitimate criticism for the book.

"I hope you have a use for the pulp from all of these juices," he stated. "So many of the juice books already out don't seem to address this problem, and that really bothers me, because the best part of the juice is being discarded, namely the fiber material left behind."

I reassured Lendon that I had already given that matter much thought. After carefully reviewing a dozen or more name-brand juice machines on the market, I had finally decided to give major emphasis to the Vita-Mix unit, "simply because it's the only one that incorporates the pulp with the juice!" Even with this, I intended to include a short section in the back on uses for the pulp for those with conventional centrifugal or masticating juicers.

"That's good! That's good!" he exclaimed with his typical college-kid enthusiasm. "That's so important for people to know, and I'm glad it's being done for a change. That will definitely enhance the value of your book even more!"

The first thing a number of fruit and vegetable pulps can be used for are as external poultices for different health problems. Some sulphur-based pulps, most notably cabbage, kale, and onion, make ideal dressings for serious burn injuries and can be changed every few hours. The sulphur helps to disinfect the injury and promote rapid tissue regeneration if the burn isn't too extensive or deep.

Carrot, cucumber, pumpkin and squash pulps are excellent for skin inflammations, due either to particular ailments like eczema, psoriasis or shingles, or else to sunburn. They exert a very cooling effect and are, therefore, also quite beneficial in fevers when placed upon the forehead, chest, and abdomen.

Other kinds of pulp have tremendous drawing properties to them. This is especially so with starchy vegetables and some fruits. In cases of diabetic leg ulcers, open sores, gangrenous wounds, lanced cysts or boils, or similar skin eruptions, the applications of potato, turnip, or rutabaga pulps will prove most efficacious indeed. In instances where there is an external tumor, such as in the case of breast cancer, where it can be carefully lanced with a sharp, sterile object, a poultice of fig pulp will draw out infection like you wouldn't believe!

Another class of pulps from very acidic or "puckering" produce that makes your mouth draw together very quickly, are valuable for knitting together cuts, scrapes, and wounds. I've seen some folk healers in Cairo, Egypt use persimmon pulp to draw the skin together in knife cuts quite effectively. These same acid pulps are equally effective for stopping bleeding.

Certain acidic pulps also help to tighten loose skin and get rid of wrinkles, when employed as facial masks. A few very expensive European health salons offer such "fruit masks" of citrus pulps to help older women get rid of distressful crow's feet around their eyes, sagging jowels on their cheeks, and loose skin on their throats. Afterwards, different plant oils such as avocado, olive, and a few nut oils are then gently massaged into the skin in a circular motion, once it has been thoroughly cleansed and prepared for this next step.

Pulps also have creative appeal for culinary needs. Some pulps with flavor to them can be worked into conventional salads like bean, carrot, cole slaw, or potato with surprising results. Try to match up things which will fit with each item: onion pulp with bean salad; grape-raisin or pineapple pulps with carrot salad; carrot, fig-date, apple, currant, and celery pulps for extravagant slaw; radish, romaine lettuce, mustard greens, or watercress pulps with potato salad. By experimenting around for a while, you should be able to come up with your own fanciful combinations that will not only taste exciting, but definitely prove you have an imaginative flair for the unusual! It's all a matter of knowing which produce items fit with each other and are digestibly and nutritionally compatible with each other. An arrangement like orange pulp with tomato salad wouldn't be agreeable, though.

Certain fruit and vegetable pulps high in natural sugar contents, are ideal for making fruit leather. These pulps can be evenly spread out on a foil-lined cookie sheet, conveniently dried in the sun or fruit drier, and then cut into various thin lengths and widths to serve as nutritious snacks later on when you're out hiking, camping, or vacationing somewhere. I've watched some of the Southwestern tribes in Arizona and New Mexico make such "fruit pemmican," which kept for months and served as delicious snacks in the wintertime.

Another way of using juice pulp is in quick breads. The following two recipes are versatile enough to handle a wide variety of fruit or vegetable pulps. In addition, they are hypoallergenic and contain no corn, egg, or milk, so food sensitive people can readily use them, depending, of course, on the kinds of pulps being used to which there are no adverse reactions.

In the first recipe, just about any type of fruit juice pulp can be employed. The other ingredients remain standard, irrespective of the fruit pulp being used.

Fresh Fruit Pulp Loaf
1/2 cup firmly packed brown sugar
1/4 cup safflower oil
1/4 cup honey or molasses
2 tablespoons sherry
1 teaspoon Golden Pride/Rawleigh pure vanilla extract
2 tablespoons baking soda
3 cups any type fresh fruit juice pulp
1 1/2 cups chopped, fresh nuts
1/2 cup dehulled sunflower seeds
2 cups sifted unbleached flour
1/2 teaspoon salt
1/4 teaspoon cinnamon
1/4 teaspoon nutmeg

Combine the brown sugar, oil, honey, sherry, and vanilla in a large mixing bowl. Mix the fruit pulp with the baking soda and then add the nuts. Combine this with the brown sugar mixture. Sift together the remaining dry ingredients and blend into fruit pulp mixture. Next turn into a greased and floured 9 × 5-inch loaf pan. Bake at 350°F. for 1 hour and 25 minutes, or until a toothpick inserted in the center of the loaf comes out clean. Permit to cool in pan about 3 minutes. Turn loaf out onto a wire rack to finish cooling. Yields one loaf that gives about 18–20 slices.

The next recipe is good for any of the squashes (including pumpkin) and starchy tubers such as potatoes, rutabagas, parsnip, and turnips. All of these vegetable juice pulps can be used with equal satisfaction. I've elected to use pumpkin pulp here, but this is only an example. Any squash or starchy tuber pulp can be substituted.

QUICK PUMPKIN BREAD
1 cup pumpkin (or any other squash or tuber pulp)
$1/3$ cup safflower oil
$1/2$ cup honey
$1/2$ cup raisins
$1^2/3$ cups whole wheat pastry flour
$1/4$ teaspoon salt
$1/2$ teaspoon cinnamon
$1/8$ teaspoon nutmeg
$1^1/2$ teaspoon baking soda

Combine pumpkin pulp (or any other type of related vegetable pulp), oil, and honey. In a medium-sized mixing bowl, combine the remaining ingredients. Stir the pumpkin mixture into the flour mixture and blend well. Pour into a well greased 8 x 4-inch loaf pan. Bake at 350°F. for almost an hour, or until a toothpick inserted in the center of the loaf comes out clean. Turn out onto a wire rack to cool. Yields one loaf that provides 16 slices.

I might mention here that even though you may have some other type of juicing machine that turns out pulp for you, it still would be a good idea to invest in a Vita-Mix unit. You can use it for mixing purposes in recipes like this and save yourself some of the arduous and time-consuming manual labor involved.

Some fruit pulp, such as apple, pear, apricot, and peach, make delicious additions to cooked oatmeal, millet, or cream-o-wheat cereals. With a few liberal shakes of cinnamon and cardamom, this breakfast treat will be naturally sweet without the benefit of added sugar or honey.

Fruit pulp is diverse enough to make any number of interesting shakes from. Use plain yogurt, large-curd cottage cheese, or tofu as the base material into which you can whip any fruit pulp you desire to. If the pulp is a little bit on the tart side, the addition of a tablespoon of pure maple syrup or blackstrap molasses will take care of that. Finally top your concoctions with a sprinkle of granola cereal, toasted seeds, or nuts for crunch and fiber.

With some fruit pulps, you may also add a little cinnamon or nutmeg and when warmed up a bit they make tasty toppings for pancakes, waffles, french toast, crepes suzette, or English muffins.

Some tangy vegetable juice pulps can be worked into extra lean ground round to make very tempting hamburger patties. They can also be worked into stuffing for poultry, along with some fruit pulps, such as apple and orange.

And don't overlook the many nifty creations you can make with any number of flavorful fruit and vegetable juice pulps by incorporating them into jello salads. I recommend that you use the Knox Unflavored Gelatin for this and stay away from the popular JELL-O®, which isn't healthy nor good for your body.

Although I've mentioned it earlier in the text several different times, I want to remind readers here that just about all fruit or vegetable pulps can be worked back into their respective juices for gritty, grainy drinks that will actively promote movements in even the most sluggish bowels. Because they are mostly fiber in content, such pulps are potent laxatives to be sure.

Finally, if you haven't figured out what else to do with your leftover pulp, then simply turn it into compost for your next spring planting. Juice pulp makes some of the best natural fertilizer that I know of. It's up there, in fact, with decayed leaves, in terms of nitrogen content, so important for healthy soil these days.

APPENDIX THREE

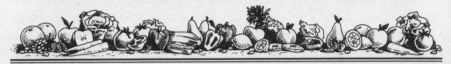

Product Suppliers and Manufacturers

As is the case with most self-improvement health books, particular products are mentioned by different authors, which they feel their readers might benefit from. Below is a list of those products and services mentioned either directly or indirectly in this book. Included are their manufacturers or suppliers, together with other pertinent information in the event some readers might want to contact them.

In no way does this imply an endorsement by the author or his publisher, only that they happen to be useful things which consumers can benefit from.

THE VITA-MIX CORPORATION
8615 Usher Rd.
Cleveland, OH 44138-9989
1-(800)-VITAMIX / (216)-235-4840

The Total Nutrition Center Whole Food Machine (Model V-S)

WAKUNAGA OF AMERICA CO., LTD.
23501 Madero
Mission Viejo, CA 92691
1-(800)-421-2998 / Calif. only 1-(800)-544-5800 /
    (714)-855-2776

Liquid Kyolic Aged Garlic Extract
Kyo-Green Chlorophyll Drink Mix

The Japanese wrote the book when it comes to superior garlic. Nothing else commercially available even holds a candle to Kyolic Garlic. In fact, Kyolic is the preferred garlic to do research with by leading scientists all over the world!

GOLDEN PRIDE/RAWLEIGH
3493 Augusta Drive
Ijamsville, MD 21754
1-(800)-864-0639 / 1-(800)-233-6550 / (301)-831-6005

Almond Extract
Banana Flavoring
Coconut Flavoring
Double Strength Vanilla
Lemon Extract
Maple Flavoring
Orange Extract
White Vanilla
Cinnamon
Ginger
Ground Cloves
Nutmeg
Formula #1, (honey, bee pollen and royal jelly liquid)
Plus K, Liquid (minerals fortification with herbs)
Formula #5, Bee Perfect (food powder)
Formula #9, Aloe Plus Drink (aloe vera, cranberry, and herb liquid)

PINES' INTERNATIONAL, INC.
P. 0. Box 1107
Lawrence, KS 66044
I-(800)-MY PINES / (913)-841-6016

Organic Red Beet Juice Powder
Rhubarb Juice Powder

I've known Ron Seibold a lot of years. He is the quintessential product of America's farming heartland and built his company on this wholesome philosophy and goodness.

FRIEDA'S BY MAIL
P. 0. Box 58488
Los Angeles, CA 90058
1-(800)-241-1771 / 1-(800)-421-9744 / (213)-627-2981

Frieda Caplan and her family specialize in supplying consumers
with hard-to-find and exotic fruits and vegetables from around
the world. She was the first person to introduce the fuzzy,
brown-skinned kiwi fruit to America in 1962. She figures it took
almost two decades for the kiwifruit to finally catch on.

RED COOPER
Route 3, Box 10
Alamo, Texas 78516-2576
1-(800)-876-4733

This company specializes in ripe, juicy citrus fruits, delicious
and exotic figs and dates from the Near East, and other delightful
fruit and fruit juice products.

OLD SOUTHWEST TRADING CO.
P. 0. Box 7545
Albuquerque, New Mexico 87194
1-(800)-748-2861

Jeffrey and Nancy Gerlach specialize in just one thing: chile
peppers. They have all types to choose from for juicing purposes—either very mild or hot enough to blow your lips plumb
off your face!

SHEPHERD'S GARDEN SEEDS
30 Irene Street
Torrington, Connecticut 06790
(203)-482-3638

This decade-old company carries seeds to some of the finest,
tastiest and juiciest vegetables around. They are well-worth
exploring in the event you wish to grow your own. They have
these vegetable seeds in stock: Artichoke, Beans (String), Beets,
Broccoli, Brussels Sprouts, Cabbage, Carrots, Cauliflower, Celery, Chard (Swiss), Cress (Water), Cucumbers, Dandelion
(French), Eggplant, Endive, Escarole, Kale, Kohlrabi, Leeks,

Lettuce, Melons, Mustard Greens, Onions, Oriental Vegetables and Greens, Parsley, Peas, Peppers (Chile and Sweet), Pumpkins, Purslane, Radishes (Red and Daikon), Spinach, Squash (Summer and Winter), Tomatoes, and Turnips.

NICHOLS GARDEN NURSERY
1190 North Pacific Highway
Albany, Oregon 97321-4598
(503)-928-9280

This second generation, 40+-year-old nursery is located in Oregon's famous Willamette Valley, where deep humus soils and mild climates have combined to bring about the best possible growing conditions. What seeds Shepherd's doesn't have, Nichols will.

TALK AMERICA
60 York Street, Suite 201
Portland, Maine 04101
1-(800)-245-CURE (2873) / (207)-775-5007

"Dr. Heinerman's Healthy Prescriptions" (A six-hour personal home study course with audio tapes and workbook. Including a free "Special Report: 50 Herbs That Can Save Your Life" with every purchase. Study course covers: "The Cave Man Diet Program" (a prehistoric way of losing weight and keeping it off for good); "Double the Power of Your Immune System" (specific programs for many immune-related diseases); and "The Management of Pain" (simple in-home chiropractic and foot-hand massage techniques, along with appropriate foods and herbs, for quick relief.)

ANTHROPOLOGICAL RESEARCH CENTER
P. O. Box 11471
Salt Lake City, UT 84147
1-(801)-521-8824

Folk Medicine Journal (An alternative health care periodical published quarterly and edited by Dr. Heinerman. Subscription rates: $30 per year (U.S. and Canada); $45 per year (foreign.))

Rex's Wheat Germ Oil (A pure vitamin E oil used by veterinarians as a food supplement for animals. It is an ideal source for youthful energy and skin. $65 for 6 month supply.)

APPENDIX FOUR

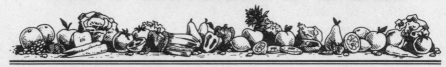

Related Reading Materials on Juicing

Editors of the University of California at Berkeley Wellness Letter. WELLNESS SHAKES AND JUICE BAR DRINKS (New York Time-Life Books, 1989), 60 pages.

Cherie Calbom and Maureen Keane. JUICING FOR LIFE (Garden City Park, NY: Avery Publishing Group, Inc., 1992), 351 pages.

William H. Lee, Ph .D . THE BOOK OF RAW FRUIT AND VEGETABLE JUICES AND DRINKS (New Canaan, CT: Keats Publishing, Inc., 1982), 177 pages.

William H. Lee, Ph.D. GETTING THE BEST OUT OF YOUR JUICER (New Canaan, CT: Keats Publishing, Inc., 1992), 175 pages.

John B. Lust. RAW JUICE THERAPY (London: Thorson's Publishers, Ltd., February 1961), 173 pages.

Gary and Shelly Null. THE JOY OF JUICING RECIPE GUIDE (New York: Golden Health Publishing, 1992), 234 pages.

APPENDIX FIVE

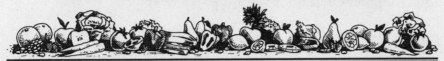

Flavorful Juice Drink Recipes

The many juice drink recipes mentioned in this section come from several different sources. My gratitude is, first of all, given to Rose Wride, Director of Home Economics at the Vita-Mix Corporation, Cleveland, Ohio for her kind assistance in making sure the recipes turned out correctly. To her test kitchen staff who tested, tasted and approved all recipes before publication. My thanks to the Vita-Mix Corporation for the extensive use of a number of recipes from their Vita-Mix *Total Nutrition Center Recipes and Instructions* book. I would also like to express my appreciation to Bernice Watson of Palo Alto, California and Marjorie Trump of Philadelphia, Pennsylvania for their original and innovative juice ideas. Finally, by my own hand have I proven the tastefulness of some of these recipes which, I guarantee, won't be found in any other book! Bon appetit and happy guzzling!

BLENDER JUICING IS ONE-STEP PROCESSING

You will notice the simple instructions which follow each recipe. Blender juicing is an easy and delightful process once you understand the basics.

Liquid and soft foods go into the blender first, followed by solid foods and ice. This should prevent the blender from stalling when it is turned on, and will allow the mixture to freely circulate until smooth. It is not necessary to blend food in steps, nor is mincing or chopping food before it is placed in the blender required. Cutting the food into one-inch pieces is usually all that is needed.

Though the following recipes can be made in any durable blender, the degree of smoothness, intensity of flavor, the speed in processing, and overall quality of juice is far superior in a Vita-Mix Total Nutrition Center.

FRUIT DRINKS

FRUIT ENERGIZER
$^1\!/_2$ ripe banana, peeled
$^1\!/_2$ cup strawberries
$^1\!/_2$ cup pineapple chunks
$^1\!/_2$ medium orange, peeled
$^1\!/_2$ medium apple, cut in half
$^1\!/_2$ teaspoon ground cinnamon
$^1\!/_2$ cup ice cubes

Place all ingredients in a blender container in the order listed. Secure lid. Blend on HIGH speed until smooth. Serve immediately.
   Yield: 2 cups

PEACHY CHERRY JUICE
$1^1\!/_2$ cups apple juice
3 peaches (or 3 cups canned)
$^1\!/_4$ cup pitted cherries
1 cup ice cubes

Place all ingredients in a blender container in the order listed. Secure lid. Blend on HIGH speed until smooth. Serve immediately.
   Yield: $4^1\!/_2$ cups

HUNZA APRICOT PICK-ME-UP
$^1\!/_2$ cup goat milk (or skim)
$^1\!/_2$ teaspoon pure vanilla extract
$^1\!/_4$ cup dried apricots, soaked in 1 cup apple juice
$^1\!/_4$ cup green seedless grapes
1 tablespoon shredded coconut
1 tablespoon raisins
1 tablespoon sunflower seeds
1 tablespoon wheat germ
$^1\!/_4$ teaspoon powdered cardamon
1 cup ice cubes

Place all ingredients in a blender container in the order listed. Secure lid. Blend on HIGH speed until smooth. Serve immediately.

Yield: 1²/₃ cups

APRICOT FLING

¹/₂ teaspoon rum extract
¹/₄ cup orange juice
¹/₄ cup lemon juice
¹/₄ cup apricot nectar
¹/₂ tablespoon lime juice
¹/₄ cup dried apricots, soaked in ¹/₂ cup apple juice
³/₄ cup ice cubes

Place all ingredients in a blender container in the order listed. Secure lid. Blend on HIGH speed until smooth. Serve immediately.

Yield: 1¹/₃ cups
Cook's Note: If desired, dilute with ice or water.

APRICOT SURPRISE

¹/₄ cup pineapple juice
¹/₄ cup ginger ale
¹/₄ teaspoon rum extract
¹/₂ orange, peeled
¹/₄ cup dried apricots, soaked in 1 cup apple juice
¹/₂ cup strawberries, frozen
¹/₂ cup ice cubes

Place all ingredients in a blender container in the order listed. Secure lid. Blend on HIGH speed until smooth. Serve immediately.

Yield: 2¹/₃ cups

BANANA-CAROB SMOOTHIE

¹/₂ cup goat milk (or skim)
¹/₂ cup soy milk powder
1 ripe banana, peeled
2 tablespoons carob powder
2 tablespoons honey
2 cups ice cubes

Place all ingredients in a blender container in the order listed. Secure lid. Blend on HIGH speed until smooth. Serve immediately.

Yield: 2²/₃ cups

ORANGE BANANA DRINK

2 oranges, peeled and quartered
1 ripe banana, peeled

Honey to taste (optional)
1 cup ice cubes

Place all ingredients in a blender in the order listed. Secure lid. Blend on HIGH speed until smooth. Serve immediately.
Yield: 2 cups

BANANA-FIG-DATE-YOGURT SHAKE

1 cup apple juice
$1/2$ teaspoon pure almond extract
$1/2$ cup plain yogurt
3 ripe bananas, peeled and broken in half
$1/4$ cup pitted dates
$1/4$ cup figs
2 tablespoons unsweetened coconut flakes
$1/2$ teaspoon powdered cardamon
2 cups ice cubes

Place all ingredients in a blender container in the order listed. Secure lid. Blend on HIGH speed until smooth. Serve immediately.
Yield: $4^1/3$ cups

PEACH BANANA ALMOND SMOOTHIE

2 tablespoons skim milk
$1/2$ medium banana, peeled
$1/8$ teaspoon almond extract
$1^1/2$ teaspoons oat bran
1 tablespoon honey
$1/4$ cup peaches, frozen
$1/2$ cup ice cubes

Place all ingredients in a blender container in the order listed. Secure lid. Blend on HIGH speed until smooth. Serve immediately.
Yield: 1 cup

BLACKBERRY SOUR

$1/4$ cup grapefruit juice
$1/2$ cup mineral water, chilled
1 tablespoon lemon juice
$1/2$ cup blackberries
1 cup ice cubes

Place all ingredients in a blender container in the order listed. Secure lid. Blend on HIGH speed until smooth. Serve immediately.
Yield: $1^1/2$ cups

BLUEBERRY FIG AND DATE SHAKE
2 cups goat milk (or skim)
2 tablespoons lemon juice
1 tablespoon pure maple syrup
1/2 teaspoon ground cinnamon
1/2 cup pitted dates
1/4 cup figs
1 cup frozen blueberries

Place all ingredients in a blender container in the order listed. Secure lid. Blend on HIGH speed until smooth. Serve immediately.
Yield: 3 1/2 cups

CRANBERRY BREEZE
1/2 cup pineapple juice, chilled
1/4 cup mineral water, chilled
1/4 cup cranberry sauce
1/4 cranberries
1/4 cup raspberries
1 cup ice cubes

Place all ingredients in a blender container in the order listed. Secure lid. Blend on HIGH speed until smooth. Serve immediately.
Yield: 2 1/2 cups
Cook's Note: Juice is very tart. If desired, sweeten to taste with honey.

APPLE-BERRY-BANANA SHAKE
1/2 cup goat milk (or skim)
1/4 teaspoon pure lemon extract
1 ripe banana, peeled
2 apples, washed and quartered
1/4 cup strawberries, frozen
1/2 cup ice cubes

Place all ingredients in a blender container in the order listed. Secure lid. Blend on HIGH speed until smooth. Serve immediately.
Yield: 3 1/2 cups

CANTALOUPE WAKEUP
1 cup cantaloupe, peeled and cut in chunks, chilled
1/2 cup watermelon chunks, seeded, chilled
1 medium orange, peeled and quartered
1 teaspoon lime juice

Place all ingredients in a blender container in the order listed.
Secure lid. Blend on HIGH speed until smooth. Serve immediately.
   Yield: 1$\frac{1}{2}$ cups

CANTALOUPE PINEAPPLE AND BANANA COOLER
$\frac{1}{2}$ cup cranberry juice
$\frac{1}{2}$ cup cantaloupe
$\frac{1}{2}$ cup pineapple, with juice, chilled
$\frac{1}{2}$ medium banana, peeled
$\frac{1}{8}$-inch slice lemon, with peel
1 tablespoon honey
$\frac{3}{4}$ cup ice cubes

Place all ingredients in a blender container in the order listed.
Secure lid. Blend on HIGH speed until smooth. Serve immediately.
   Yield: 2$\frac{1}{2}$ cups

STRAWBERRY-KIWI CORDIAL
2$\frac{1}{4}$ cups orange juice
1 medium kiwi fruit, peeled and halved
1 cup strawberries
1 cup ice cubes

Place all ingredients in a blender container in the order listed.
Secure lid. Blend on HIGH speed until smooth. Serve immediately.
   Yield: 3$\frac{1}{2}$ cups

GRAPE-RAISIN SPRITZER
1 cup pineapple juice, chilled
1 cup mineral water, chilled
2 cups green seedless grapes
$\frac{1}{2}$ cup raisins, soaked in enough pineapple juice to cover

Place all ingredients in a blender container in the order listed.
Secure lid. Blend on HIGH speed until smooth. Serve immediately.
   Yield: 4 cups

RASPBERRY WATERMELON COOLER
3 cups watermelon (seeded)
1 cup frozen strawberries
Place all ingredients in a blender container in the order listed.
Secure lid. Blend on HIGH speed until smooth. Serve immediately.
   Yield: 2$\frac{1}{2}$ cups

GRAPEFRUIT COMBO

$^1/_4$ pink or red grapefruit, peeled
$^1/_2$ orange, peeled and cut in half
$^1/_3$ cup pineapple, chilled
$^1/_2$ cup white or red seedless grapes
1 cup ice cubes

Place all ingredients in a blender container in the order listed. Secure lid. Blend on HIGH speed until smooth. Serve immediately.
Yield: $2^1/_2$ *cups*

ALCOHOL-FREE GRAPE DAIQUIRI

$^1/_2$ teaspoon rum extract
$^1/_4$ cup grape juice
1 tablespoon frozen grape juice concentrate
$^1/_4$ cup red seedless grapes
$^1/_4$ cup green seedless grapes
$^1/_4$ cup blue seedless grapes

Place all ingredients in a blender container in the order listed. Secure lid. Blend on HIGH speed until smooth. Serve immediately.
Yield: $1^3/_4$ *cups*

ALCOHOL-FREE CITRUS SANGRIA

$^3/_4$ cup white grape juice
2 cups mineral water, chilled
1 cup canned pineapple, with juice
1 lemon, peeled and quartered
1 lime, peeled and quartered
1 ruby-red grapefruit, peeled and quartered

Place all ingredients in a blender container in the order listed. Secure lid. Blend on HIGH speed until smooth. Serve immediately.
Yield: *6 cups*

PINEAPPLE BACHELOR PLUS TWO

$^1/_4$ cup fresh pineapple
$^1/_2$ orange, peeled
$^1/_2$ tangerine, peeled
1-inch slice apple
$^1/_2$ ripe banana, peeled
1 teaspoon pure maple syrup
1 teaspoon dark honey
$^1/_2$ cup ice cubes

Place all ingredients in a blender container in the order listed.
Secure lid. Blend on HIGH speed until smooth. Serve immediately.

Yield: 1¹/₂ cups

MANGO SURPRISE

¹/₄ cup pineapple juice, chilled
¹/₂ cup fresh or canned pineapple, chilled
¹/₂ ripe banana, peeled
¹/₂ cup mango slices, peeled
¹/₄ cup strawberries, frozen
1 orange, peeled and quartered
¹/₂ cup ice cubes

Place all ingredients in a blender container in the order listed.
Secure lid. Blend on HIGH speed until smooth. Serve immediately.

Yield: 2¹/₂ cups

MIXED FRUIT SMOOTHIE

¹/₂ cup plain yogurt
1 ripe banana
¹/₂ orange, peeled and cut in half
¹/₄ cup peaches, frozen
¹/₂ cup frozen strawberries, sweetened
¹/₄ cup ice cubes

Place all ingredients in a blender container in the order listed.
Secure lid. Blend on HIGH speed until smooth. Serve immediately.

Yield: 2¹/₂ cups

STRAWBERRY GRAPE JUICE

1 cup frozen strawberries
1 cup white seedless grapes
1 cup red seedless grapes
¹/₂ cup ice cubes

Place all ingredients in a blender container in the order listed.
Secure lid. Blend on HIGH speed until smooth. Serve immediately.

Yield: 2¹/₂ cups

VEGETABLE DRINKS

TOMATO GAZPACHO

3 cups tomato juice
¹/₃ cup red wine vinegar
¹/₂ cup Rex's® Wheat Germ Oil

Dash Tabasco sauce
1 teaspoon liquid Kyolic® Aged Garlic Extract
2 large ripe tomatoes, quartered
1 cucumber, peeled and cut in 1-inch pieces
1 small onion, quartered
1 sweet green bell pepper (seeds intact), quartered
Granulated kelp, to taste

Place all ingredients in a blender container in the order listed. Secure lid. Blend on HIGH speed until smooth. Serve immediately.

Yield: 3 cups

SPICY SQUASH SHAKE

1 cup goat milk
1 1/2 tablespoons molasses
1/2 cup butternut squash, cooked then chilled
4 teaspoons tofu
Pinch of ground cardamom
Pinch of ground mace
Pinch of ground nutmeg

Place all ingredients in a blender container in the order listed. Secure lid. Blend on HIGH speed until smooth. Serve immediately.

Yield: 1 1/2 cups

SPINACH COCKTAIL

1 teaspoon liquid Kyolic® Aged Garlic Extract
1 cup chilled tomato juice
1 cup strong peppermint tea, cold
1 cup fresh spinach leaves
1 cup ice cubes

Place all ingredients in a blender container in the order listed. Secure lid. Blend on HIGH speed until smooth. Serve immediately.

Yield: 2 1/2 cups

CHILI PEPPER COMBO

1 cup tomato juice
1 cup romaine lettuce

COOK'S NOTE

See Appendix section under Wakunaga of America for obtaining Kyolic® Aged Garlic Extract and Kyo-Green® Powder, two of America's premier health food products.

1 purple cabbage leaf
2-inch slice of carrot
1 tablespoon sweet Vidalia onion
1 teaspoon parsley
1/4 cup sweet red or green bell pepper
1/2 teaspoon pimiento
Pinch of cayenne pepper
1/8 teaspoon Tabasco sauce
1/2 teaspoon Worcestershire sauce
1/2 teaspoon liquid Kyolic® Aged Garlic Extract
1 cup ice cubes

Place all ingredients in a blender container in the order listed. Secure lid. Blend on HIGH speed until smooth. Serve immediately.
Yield: 2 cups

BUTTERMILK AND CUCUMBER REFRESHER
1 cup buttermilk
2-inch cucumber slice, peeled
4 small peppermint leaves
2 ice cubes

Place all ingredients in a blender container in the order listed. Secure lid. Blend on HIGH speed until smooth. Serve immediately.
Yield: 1 cup

CUCUMBER COOLER
1/2 cup lowfat sour cream or plain yogurt
1 cup cucumber, peeled and cut into 1-inch pieces
Pinch of granulated kelp
1 tablespoon fresh onion
1/2 cup ice cubes

Place all ingredients in a blender container in the order listed. Secure lid. Blend on HIGH speed until smooth. Serve immediately.
Yield: 1 1/2 cups

SAUERKRAUT WITH BEET
1/2 cup sauerkraut juice
1/2 cup sauerkraut
1/4 cup canned beets
1 teaspoon Kyo-Green® Powder
1 cup ice cubes

Place all ingredients in a blender container in the order listed. Secure lid. Blend on HIGH speed until smooth. Serve immediately.
Yield: 1¹/₂ cups

CARROT BEET DELIGHT
1¹/₂ cups mineral water, chilled
1 cup carrot juice
1 cup goat milk (or skim)
¹/₂ cup beets
1 cup ice cubes

Place all ingredients in a blender container in the order listed. Secure lid. Blend on HIGH speed until smooth. Serve immediately.
Yield: 3³/₄ cups

TRIATHLON BEET DRINK
1 cup carrot juice
1 cup sweet green bell pepper, cut in 1-inch pieces
¹/₂ cup beets

Place all ingredients in a blender container in the order listed. Secure lid. Blend on HIGH speed until smooth. Serve immediately.
Yield: 1¹/₂ cups

MIXED VEGETABLE-CAULIFLOWER TONIC
1¹/₂ cups carrot juice
2 cups cauliflower, steamed and chilled
2 celery ribs, with leaves
1 teaspoon Pine's® Beet Juice Powder Concentrate
1 teaspoon Pine's® Rhubarb Juice Powder Concentrate
1 teaspoon Kyo-Green® Powder
¹/₂ clove garlic

Place all ingredients in a blender container in the order listed. Secure lid. Blend on HIGH speed until smooth. Serve immediately.
Yield: 2 cups

HORSERADISH SALUTE
³/₄ cup carrot juice
1 teaspoon tomato juice
1 teaspoon sauerkraut juice
2 tablespoons horseradish sauce
2 radishes

Place all ingredients in a blender container in the order listed. Secure lid. Blend on HIGH speed until smooth. Serve immediately.

Yield: 1 cup

TERIYAKI TOMATO JUICE
1/2 cup canned tomatoes or *tomato juice*
1/2 cup celery, with leaves
2 tablespoons sweet green bell pepper
1/3 cup carrots
2 tablespoons onion
2 tablespoons Teriyaki sauce
1 teaspoon liquid Kyolic® Aged Garlic Extract
1 teaspoon Kyo-Green® Powder
1 1/2 cups ice cubes

Place all ingredients in a blender container in the order listed. Secure lid. Blend on HIGH speed until smooth. Serve immediately.

Yield: 3 cups

GREEN VEGGIE COCKTAIL
1/2 cup nonfat sour cream or *plain yogurt*
1/2 cup cucumber, peeled
1/4 cup broccoli
1/2 cup peas, frozen or fresh, steamed and chilled
1/4 cup onion
1 teaspoon liquid Kyolic® Aged Garlic Extract
1 teaspoon Kyo-Green® Powder
1/2 cup ice cubes

Place all ingredients in a blender container in the order listed. Secure lid. Blend on HIGH speed until smooth. Serve immediately.

Yield: 1 1/2 cups

CARROT JUICE PLUS
1 cup mineral water, chilled
1 1/2 cups carrots, cut in 1-inch pieces
1 teaspoon Kyo-Green® Powder
1 cup ice cubes

Place all ingredients in a blender container in the order listed. Secure lid. Blend on HIGH speed until smooth. Serve immediately.

Yield: 2 cups

BRUSSELS SPROUTS BON APPETIT
1 cup tomato juice
1 cup carrot juice

1 cup celery, with leaves
4 Brussels sprouts, raw
1 teaspoon granulated kelp
1 cup ice cubes

Place all ingredients in a blender container in the order listed. Secure lid. Blend on HIGH speed until smooth. Serve immediately.
Yield: 3$\frac{1}{2}$ cups

HOT VEGETABLE DRINKS

COOK'S CAUTION

In preparing any of the Hot Vegetable Drinks if you are not using a Vita-Mix, scalding may result. It is important that you start with *cool* ingredients. Blend smooth and heat to desired temperature in a double boiler.

GARLIC-ONION HOT TODDY
4 cups mineral water, boiling
3 tablespoons tomato paste
1 medium carrot, cut in 1-inch pieces
1 rib celery, with leaves
2 to 3 green onions
5 bouillon cubes
1 tablespoon liquid Kyolic® Aged Garlic Extract

Place all ingredients in a blender container in the order listed. Secure lid. Blend on HIGH speed until smooth. Serve immediately.
Yield: 4 cups

SWEET PEA SOUP DRINK
1 cup chicken, ham or vegetable stock, boiling
1 teaspoon liquid Kyolic® Aged Garlic Extract
$\frac{1}{2}$ cup frozen peas, thawed
1-inch slice sweet red bell pepper
1 to 2-inch slice carrot
Dash of black pepper
Dash of oregano
Pinch of granulated kelp

Place all ingredients in a blender container in the order listed. Secure lid. Blend on HIGH speed until smooth. Serve immediately.
Yield: 1$\frac{1}{2}$ cups

SWEET PEAS AND TATORS

1 cup skim milk, hot
¹/₄ cup nonfat sour cream substitute or *plain yogurt*
¹/₂ cup sweet peas (fresh or frozen), steamed
¹/₂ cup potatoes, peeled and cooked
1 teaspoon onion
¹/₄ to ¹/₂ teaspoon chicken bouillon (optional)
¹/₂ teaspoon Kyo-Green® Powder

Place all ingredients in a blender container in the order listed.
Secure lid. Blend on HIGH speed until smooth. Serve immediately.
Yield: 1¹/₂ cups

HOT PEAS BROCCOLI AND ASPARAGUS

¹/₂ cup peas, fresh or *frozen, steamed*
¹/₂ cup broccoli, steamed
¹/₄ cup fresh asparagus, steamed
1 tablespoon onion
¹/₄ teaspoon chicken bouillon (optional)
¹/₂ cup chicken broth, hot
1 tablespoon lowfat cheddar cheese

Place all ingredients in a blender container in the order listed.
Secure lid. Blend on HIGH speed until smooth. Serve immediately.
Yield: 1¹/₂ cups

FRUIT FOR BABY

APRICOT-APPLE BABY FOOD

1 cup goat milk
1 medium apple, peeled and quartered
1 cup apricots, fresh or canned

Place all ingredients in a blender container in the order listed.
Secure lid. Blend on HIGH speed until smooth. Serve immediately.
Yield: 1³/₄ cups

ORANGE AND APPLE FOR BABY

1 medium orange, peeled and quartered
1 medium apple, peeled and quartered
¹/₃ cup mineral water

Place all ingredients in a blender container in the order listed.
Secure lid. Blend on HIGH speed until smooth. Serve immediately.
Yield: 1 cup

PEAR-ORANGE DRINK FOR BABY
1 cup orange juice, chilled
1 pear, quartered

Place all ingredients in a blender container in the order listed. Secure lid. Blend on HIGH speed until smooth. Serve immediately.
Yield: $1^1/_2$ cups

PEACH BANANA FOR BABY
$^1/_2$ teaspoon lemon juice
$^3/_4$ cup goat milk
1 medium banana, peeled
$^1/_2$ cup fresh or canned peaches
1 date, pitted

Place all ingredients in a blender container in the order listed. Secure lid. Blend on HIGH speed until smooth. Serve immediately.
Yield: $1^2/_3$ cups

Cook's Note: Mixture becomes pudding-like as it sets.

VEGETABLES FOR BABY

STRING BEANS AND BARLEY FOR BABY
$^1/_2$ cup string beans, cooked
$^1/_4$ cup soybean milk (reconstituted)
1 teaspoon Gerber's® barley cereal

Place all ingredients in a blender container in the order listed. Secure lid. Blend on HIGH speed until smooth. Serve immediately.
Yield: $^1/_2$ cup

GARDEN PEAS FOR BABY
1 cup goat milk (or skim)
2 teaspoons Gerber's® barley cereal
$^3/_4$ cup cooked peas

Place all ingredients in a blender container in the order listed. Secure lid. Blend on HIGH speed until smooth. Serve immediately.
Yield: 1 cup

CARROT JUICE FOR BABY
$^3/_4$ cup carrot juice
1 cup goat milk

Place all ingredients in a blender container in the order listed. Secure lid. Blend on HIGH speed until smooth. Serve immediately.
Yield: 1³/₄ cups

COOK'S NOTE

Any of the baby food recipes may also be given to those who are recuperating from long-term illness or surgery or simply those elderly who cannot handle solid foods.

INDEX